EMERGENCY CARE

FOR BEGINNERS

BRANDA NURT

Table of Contents

EMERGENCY CARE FOR BEGINNERS
How to Handle Insect and Animal Bites

EMERGENCY CARE FOR BEGINNERS
How to Handle A Broken Bone

EMERGENCY CARE FOR BEGINNERS
How to Heal Someone Who Has Been Shot

EMERGENCY CARE

FOR BEGINNERS

How to Handle Insect and Animal Bites

BRANDA NURT

Introduction

An insect or animal bite can be mild, extremely unpleasant, or deadly. Knowing what to do in an emergency is going to be the difference between life or death. Whether you are alone or with another person, you need to know how to handle an insect or animal bite. There are items you should carry in your first aid kit on a hike, in your car, or even at home. Furthermore, you should be aware of the types of insects or animals that are dangerous in your area or where you are traveling too, to ensure you have the proper items on hand.

A female, age 39, was recently bitten by a spider. Living in the Colorado mountains, this spider could have been one of a few poisonous spiders, including a brown recluse. It happened during the night, while the person was sleeping, so the spider went unidentified. However, the reaction did not go unnoticed. At first, an innocent-looking zit appeared on the chin, but after examining the area, it was clearly not a large pimple. The chin started swelling, with pain radiating down the left side of the chin and neck. A few days later, the skin started to appear like a scab in the center of the wound. Necropsy was a concern, a medical condition where the skin dies due to the toxic venom of a spider. Typically, such things happen with a brown recluse bite, but other spiders can cause the same reaction.

Thankfully, a little ointment helped stop the necrosis, but it did leave a small scar on the chin. The treatment for the reaction to the spider bite required antibiotics. Unfortunately, the chosen antibiotic was made with a sulfa component, like shellfish. Two weeks went by, and on the night of the last dose of antibiotics, the woman broke out in a full-body rash, finally showing an allergic reaction to the antibiotic.

When a new antibiotic is used, a person may not present with an allergic reaction until the dose is completed; mainly, if the allergy is mild or other medications are being used, such as allergy medication. The patient had to get a steroid shot and take a daily dose of antihistamine.

This account is provided to help you understand that sometimes the initial treatment or the mild bite can become something much more significant and risk a person's health, even a day or two weeks after the incident. Your first aid steps during an insect or animal bite can determine the future for the person you are helping, even if it is yourself.

The following guide will be split into three parts:

1. Creating a First Aid Kit

2. Insect

3. Animals

Each section will discuss some of the worst insects or animals that you could encounter and the emergency care you should administer. Please note each person is different in physiology, meaning size, allergies, and reactions, so while these steps are provided, professional emergency medical care should be provided as quickly as possible.

Note: If you're in a life-threatening or emergency medical situation, seek medical assistance immediately.

SECTION 1

First Aid and
CPR Equipment

Being prepared for any emergency is essential. While the main focus of this book is to provide you with immediate emergency medical care procedures for an insect or animal bite, you still need to be prepared for any situation you might encounter. This section will outline what you should carry with you in your car, in your hiking backpack, or when you travel.

Traveling to different regions of the world can put you in danger from different animals and insects. For example, the United States has only one lethal scorpion, while the Middle East and Africa have several species.

Chapter 1

First Aid Kit

Building your first aid kits is simple. You can buy a kit that comes with nearly everything you would need in case of an emergency. Depending on the size of the kit, you can have several sizes of Band-Aids, antibiotic ointment, burn cream, gauze, tweezers, and sterile syringes to help wash wounds. Survival websites and stores sell a variety of different packs. Typically, these kits do not come with anything to help with insect bites. For example, your kit probably does not have an insect bite wipe or StingEze to help stop the itch.

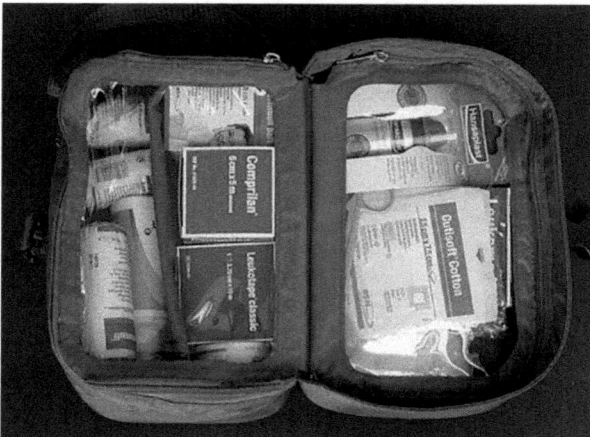

First Aid Kits are also going to lack things like an Epi-Pen because the medication requires a prescription.

The following is a list of what your kit should have for insect or animal bites:

- Multiple sizes of Band-Aids to cover a bite or open wound and prevent infection
- Gauze for larger wounds
- Splint for arms and legs for any breaks or immobilization requirements
- Antibiotic ointment to help with infection
- Alcohol wipes or sanitization syringes to clean the wounds
- Tourniquet (may be necessary for animal bites)
- Insect bite wipes to alleviate the itch (also comes in a roller device)
- Antihistamine medication
- Pain reliever
- Epi-Pen (if you or someone you travel with has a known allergy)
- Cold Pack (to help with swelling)
- Face mask (for mouth to mask resuscitation)

Most insect bites will have a mild reaction, but envenomation (the delivery of venom into prey) can be high enough to cause severe discomfort and even death depending on the insect bite or sting.

Animal bites can be the more severe issue with loss of limb, punctured artery or veins, and heart troubles due to loss of blood. You want to make sure your first aid kit has everything you need to stop blood loss or an allergic reaction.

Chapter 2

CPR Equipment and CPR

Before the new millennium, you would have found it hard to obtain certain CPR (cardiopulmonary resuscitation) equipment for emergencies In particular, you would have struggled to treat an anaphylactic (allergic) reaction or after an animal attack. Now, you can find specific equipment that will help you in an emergency by visiting a survival store, ordering online, or from a magazine.

Two things are more accessible than ever to add to your first aid kit:

- Defibrillator

- Oxygen tank

Defibrillator

A defibrillator is a device that will "shock" the heart to restart it. While AEDs are not the most inexpensive device to add to your first aid kit, a defibrillator can be the best thing you ever bring with you. Medical companies have designed the devices to be small, easy to store or carry, for those emergency medical situations where a hospital or medical center is too far to help a patient whose heart stops working.

Before you buy this equipment, you must take the First Aid and CPR course through any regulated provider such as a scuba diving company, medical center, or health center.

You also need to read the instructions thoroughly before you ever consider using it on a person. Most of these devices will cost you a few hundred dollars, but well worth it if you intend on traveling to locations where dangerous animals and insects live.

Oxygen Tank

Like the defibrillator, oxygen tanks for first aid kits have become more common and less expensive than in the past. In fact, one company makes an oxygen bottle for altitude sickness. It fits over the face and provides air to a person. It does not secure in place, which makes it hard to use when you need to provide air to an unconscious individual.

Through survival and medical supply stores, you can buy a small oxygen tank complete with an air hose and mask that will secure in place.

CPR

CPR techniques have alerted in recent years. It used to be a certain compression amount and then a breath of air. Now, people are asked to get in at least 100 compressions in sixty seconds, two breaths, and then resuming compressions when there is no heartbeat or breathing.

The following will describe the procedure; however, it is better if you sign up for a class through the Red Cross, medical center, scuba diving center. You want to ensure you are certified to provide first aid and CPR; especially, if you intend on spending a lot of time outdoors, traveling, and because it can save a life no matter the situation you might find yourself in. If Covid-19 has taught us anything, it is difficult to determine what could happen.

The Red Cross is the American authority on CPR. They offer classes in all states, and you can sign up online for a class near you. These are the steps the Red Cross requests you make:

1. Check the scene for any remaining danger, such as a scorpion still hanging around or a bear ready to continue its attack.

2. Go to the person, tap them on the shoulder and shout, "are you okay?" You need to make sure a person needs help before providing any first aid or CPR. The loud voice is to help if the person is just in shock, and it takes a moment or three for your words to get through.

3. Call 911 for emergency personnel when it is clear a person requires help. You can also have someone else on the scene make the emergency call.

4. If you have an automated external defibrillator (AED), make sure you have it handy, along with your first aid kit, and face mask.

5. For CPR to be administered, the person will need to be on their back, in a prone position.

6. Carefully roll the person, moving them as little as possible.

7. Open the airway by tilting the head back slightly to lift the chin and provide a more direct airflow.

8. Check for breathing by placing your ear near the mouth and nose. At the same time, look to see if their chest is rising and falling with breath. Listen carefully for any air for no more than 10 seconds. If there are no signs of breathing, it is time to begin resuscitation techniques.

9. Also, check for a pulse. Typically, no breathing will mean the heart has also stopped, but you want to make sure. Check for a pulse on the neck, using two fingers or using two fingers on the wrist search for a pulse. The neck is often a more natural choice because the pulse is more energetic near the jugular vein.

3-Step CPR

1. Push hard and push fast. Locate the heart between the breastbones. Place one hand flat on the area and interlock your other hand over the top. Using your body weight provides 100 compressions per minute and make sure you are pushing down at least 2 inches deep. (If you are doing CPR correctly, there is a chance that you will break rib bones around the heart.) If you have an AED, you can use it to restart the heart.

2. Deliver to rescue breaths after providing a minute of compression. Make sure the head is tilted back, and the chin is lifted slightly. Pinch the nose and place your face mask

over the mouth to create a perfect seal. You can also place your mouth over the person's mouth to make a complete seal. Blow into the person's mouth and watch for the chest to rise. Once two breaths are provided, go back to compressions.

3. Continue CPR until EMS or another trained medical responder arrives.

Never use an AED if you have not read how to use it and used it during a CPR training course. Many things can go wrong, including putting yourself in danger if you use one without the proper training. Furthermore, a person or the person's family can sue you if you administer CPR incorrectly.

Furthermore, the National Health Service, a UK organization, has a slightly different take on CPR. While they do request 100 to 120 compressions per minute and breaths, it is said that you should provide 30 compressions, provide 2 breaths, and then resume compressions for another 30. They also have a hands-only CPR where you provide compressions only and no rescue breaths.

It does not matter where you receive your training or which country provides you with certification if you remember your training during an emergency.

Tourniquets

A lot of animal bites are going to require tourniquets or bandaging to stop blood loss. Here are the steps to use a tourniquet.

1. Determine where the blood loss is happening and if it is life-threatening. Copious amounts of blood will require a tourniquet.

2. A belt or other sash like material should be wrapped around the extremity, such as a leg or arm. It needs to be higher than the wound but within an inch or two of the area.

3. Get the material as tight as possible. You may use a stick to twist the material as tight as you can get it. Blood flow stopped to an extremity can mean the removal of that limb depending on how fast medical personnel can get to the injury. However, consistent blood flow will mean death.

4. You will also want to pack the wound with gauze and wrap a bandage around it to help stop blood flow.

If the wound is on the abdomen or upper body, a tourniquet is not going to help. You will need to pack the wound with as much gauze as possible, wrap a tight bandage around the person, and continue providing gauze and bandages around the wound until you can get to medical help.

You should always stop blood flow before attempting to revive a person since the loss of blood, the shock from it can be the reason for the heart and breathing to stop.

SECTION 2

Insects

Insect bites can range from mild irritation, such as a small bump and itch, to something very life-threatening. Because bites and stings can differ among individuals, a look at how mild bites and stings can affect you or another person and the treatment to help will be discussed briefly. More details on what to do for specific insects like brown recluse spiders and black widow spiders will also be provided in this section.

Chapter 3

Mild Bites

Mild insect bites happen often, and sometimes you do not notice there is even a bump until you scratch the itch that has suddenly presented. After a few minutes, the irritation goes away. This type of bite is something that may seem innocuous, but the itch sometimes remains longer than you find comfortable. For example, fleas, flies, bees, and ants can all provide a mild bite or sting that is irritating for thirty minutes to several days.

After constant scratching, you open the wound. You could gain a mild infection because you did not think to clean the area or apply an anti-itch remedy. Here are some steps and a few home remedies you can use to address a mild insect bite and prevent infection:

1. Wash the bite area. You may not feel the bite, but a consistent itching sensation and a small welt tell you there is one. Cleaning the bite area will help prevent infection in the event the small hole caused by the bite or sting is open.

2. Apply an anti-itch product, such as StingEze or Hydrocortisone. Some products contain benzocaine and

phenol, which help relieve itching. Camphor can also be a natural ingredient that works as an antiseptic. Hydrocortisone, as the name implies, is a chemical that helps relieve itching. Such products are meant to help with bites and stings from ticks, mosquitoes, bees, ants, deerflies, fire ants, horseflies, sand fleas, and chiggers. Apply the cream to prevent yourself from scratching the bite and creating an open wound. If you do not have a first aid product on hand like StingEze, you can use natural products or vinegar. Vinegar has an analgesic that will numb the pain or itchy feeling. Simply dab a little on a cotton ball around and top of the welt.

3. Use a cold compress or cold pack to relieve swelling around the wound area.

4. Cover with an appropriately sized bandage.

5. Wash the area twice daily, apply anti-itch cream as needed, and avoid creating an open wound.

6. Monitor the welt for infection.

7. Monitor your symptoms if difficulty breathing, rash, pain, or increased swelling occur, visit a doctor.

8. If puss exudes from the wound, visit a physician.

Herbs to Relieve Mild Insect Bites

Herbs or plants, including the essential oils you can derive from the plants, are helpful to stop the itching feeling an insect bite can create.

1. Basil

2. Chamomile

3. Lavender

4. Mint

5. Rosemary

6. Tea Tree

The six plants mentioned above can be found in essential oil form, or you can take a leaf directly from the plant and apply it to an insect bite. There are over a dozen herbs and plants which can help with mild bites, including eucalyptus, pennyroyal, thyme, calendula, lemongrass, and clove.

It's a good idea to learn to identify these plants in the wild and to have some on hand at home. Mint is extremely easy to grow and can help with more than insect bites. It is known for its digestive properties, making a lovely herbal tisane, when steeped for 10 to 15 minutes in hot water. Mint can relieve stomach upset, nausea, and abdominal pain.

The above steps and tips will help with mild bites. To handle other insect bites that are more severe, keep reading.

Chapter 4

Bees and Wasps

B ee and Wasp stings can range from a mild to a severe allergic reaction, which includes anaphylaxis. Anaphylaxis is a condition where the throat closes within seconds or minutes, preventing a person from being able to breathe. The condition begins because the immune system releases chemicals into the body that can cause a person to go into shock. The blood pressure will drop, so a rapid, shallow pulse presents, along with a skin rash, nausea, and vomiting.

It is possible to treat a bee sting if you have the proper supplies in your first aid kit. However, if you have never been exposed to a bee sting or do not know if you have an allergy, it is more difficult to have specific options on hand.

Let's discuss the emergency care before getting into the difficulty of keeping some supplies on hand.

Steps to Treat a Bee Sting without an Allergic Reaction
1. Check the area of the sting.

2. A welt typically begins immediately due to the bee "venom."

3. From the welt, a rash or redness can appear.

4. Look at the point of entry for the stinger to determine if the stinger is still in the skin. A bee's stinger is 1.6 millimeters in size; however, it can break off and be smaller. With a welt, it may not be readily apparent that the stinger is in the skin and not still attached to the bee.

5. Wash the area gently.

6. Ice the area, careful of the fact that the stinger may still be in the skin. You want to alleviate the skin and stop the swelling before attempting to remove any stinger that may remain.

7. If the stinger stays in the skin, use small forceps or tweezers to pull the stinger from the welt gently. You may need a medical professional if you see a piece of the stinger but cannot grab it with tweezers.

8. Monitor the person or yourself for possible allergic reactions. If a rash present, lightheadedness, vomiting, low blood pressure, or breathing difficulties get to the nearest medical facility, quickly. You can administer liquid Benadryl to a person who is starting to show an allergic reaction to help lessen the effects and get to a medical professional.

9. Apply a topical treatment, whether it is a plant or essential oil, or a first aid product like an anti-itch wipe.

10. If you have a headache, take a pain reliever.

Depending on where the bee stings you, your reaction can be more painful. For example, a bee sting on the back of the neck can swell larger, cause extreme redness, and an intense headache without being an allergic reaction. It is due to the nerve center being so close or a "direct" hit by the bee that can temporarily cause extreme discomfort.

If there is no allergic reaction, then a combination of Benadryl or another type of analgesic and antiseptic helps reduce the pain and prevent infection of the area.

When a sting is an emergency, you must do your best with what you have on hand. There are several things you can have in your first aid kit, even if you do not know if you or someone around you has a bee allergy.

Bee Stings with an Allergic Reaction

You are going to treat someone slightly differently if they have a known allergic reaction or present with an immediate allergic reaction.

1. Grab their Epi-Pen or epinephrine pen. Epinephrine is a drug that helps with anaphylactic shock in people with severe allergies. Epi-Pen is just one brand of this medication. There are others, and if you or a family member has a severe allergy, you may have a prescription for this medication. If you do not have an allergy that requires Epinephrine or that is known, then you are not going to be able to have this remedy in your first aid kit or on your person. Administer the medication immediately if there is a known allergy!

2. Once the medication is administered, you can follow the steps above, with regards to cleaning the wound, getting itch cream, and applying ice to the welt.

3. You still need to get to an emergency care facility. The medication is meant to help save a life, but you want to have a doctor provide the "all-clear" for your allergic reaction.

Sans the Epi-Pen

A few years ago, the Epi-Pen skyrocketed in cost. Suddenly, the most used emergency answer to anaphylaxis was unreachable by most of the world's population. People with a prescription were being charged upwards of $500 just for one pen. Thankfully, there are alternatives to this brand name. GoodRx offers generic versions of the epinephrine pen that are more cost-effective.

But you still must have a prescription for such devices.

If you or someone in your family does not have a severe allergy that would require a quick shot of Epinephrine to save their life, then you will not be able to have this as part of your first aid kit.

What can you do instead? Here are some alternatives.

Providing Oxygen

The main problem with a severe allergic reaction to a bee sting is low blood pressure and restricted breathing. While it will not save a person, you can administer oxygen until you can reach emergency medical personnel who will have Epinephrine.

There are two options for oxygen.

1. Oxygen bottles meant for altitude sickness. These bottles have a mouth covering that allows you to squirt and inhale oxygen.

2. Purchasing a medical oxygen tank with a hose. This can be expensive, but at most medical supply locations, you can purchase a small, emergency oxygen tank complete with a hose for the nostrils that will administer constant oxygen to a patient through the nose and down the airway.

However, you must be overly cautious with either choice. The person may try to take shallow breaths and find their airway obstructed, even with a direct supply of oxygen. The hope is that enough air will get through the restricted passage to help keep the person alive until you can reach proper medical care.

You should only pause long enough to supply the oxygen before helping the person to medical professionals.

If the person is also experiencing a drop in blood pressure, you must lie them down and elevate their feet, so the heart does not have to work as hard to pump blood.

Again, these are quick measures before rushing a person to the emergency room to get help with the allergic reaction.

Liquid Benadryl

Another thing to have in your first aid kit is liquid Benadryl for allergies. Swallowing a tablet is not comfortable with a restricted airway; however, when symptoms present, and before the airway is completely blocked, providing liquid Benadryl can help slow the progression of symptoms.

Benadryl has properties to help with allergic reactions, including reducing inflammation. It is by no means a full solution to the problem. You still need to get the person or yourself to a medical professional to alleviate the issue altogether.

Unfortunately, with bees, it is never clear if someone has an allergy until they are stung. Once you know that you react severely, you can get a prescription for an injection of Epinephrine, to help should you get stung in the future.

Wasps

Wasp stings are remarkably similar in an allergic reaction to bees. The difference between a wasp and bee sting is the size of the stinger. Wasps have a more extended stinger that can be up to 2.5 millimeters in size.

If a sting occurs, you need to check that the stinger did not break off in the skin. Left inside, it can lead to an infection and a prolonged recovery time.

You also do not want to worsen the skin area by pulling it out without first using ice and then gently pulling with tweezers. The inflammation could hide the stinger if it broke off, which is why you need the ice to help reduce the welt.

Skin and Healing

Most times, a wound can close within 72 hours. The skin can cover over a prick by a stinger in such a brief time and leave it inside, causing problems for you. If the skin does close and the stinger is still inside, you will need to seek a medical professional who will most likely make an incision to remove the stinger and allow the wound to bleed or ooze pus.

You will know if the skin is infected from the bee or wasp sting if the welt remains for a prolonged period. Usually, when ice or a cold pack is administered within minutes of the sting, the welt will reduce in size within two to four hours. However, if the stinger is inside the welt may not reduce in size. It may not grow larger either, but it can be very painful to the touch and remain red.

Types of Bees and Wasps

There are several species of bees and a few different wasps. Knowing the diverse types can help you determine what type of sting they may provide.

African Bees: African Bees have been migrating around the world, including the United States. They are highly prevalent in Arizona, Arkansas, California, Florida, Louisiana, Nevada, New Mexico, and Texas. Many refer to African Bees as killer bees because they have caused more deaths worldwide than any other bees. It is not that their venom is more potent than

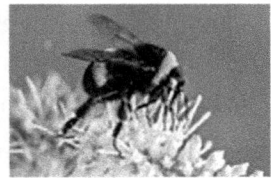

other bees. It is that they tend to swarm so a person can be stung hundreds or thousands of times.

One sting may not kill a person who is not allergic to bees; however, hundreds or thousands of stings can kill a person simply from the overabundance of venom in the body, which it is unable to fight. Quick emergency care is paramount to saving a person. If many stings occur, get to the nearest hospital immediately.

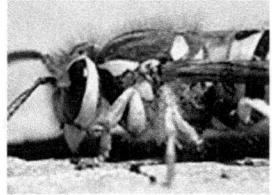

Yellow Jacket: The most common bee in the United States is known as the Yellow Jacket. It has a distinct appearance with black and yellow bands going from the waist to the bottom where the stinger is.

Bumble Bee: Bumblebees are more significant than the Yellow Jacket, and they do have yellow markings, with black underneath. The Bumblebee may look innocent, but when provoked, it can sting.

Honeybees: Honeybees are orangish-brown with a thick waist. They do have a stinger.

Umbrella Wasp: The Umbrella wasp is orangish-brown with long legs and wings. They also have a "threaded" waist with a narrow body. It is a common wasp in the higher elevations.

Bald-Face Hornet: Bald-Face hornet or wasp is mostly black with a whitish rear end.

Mud Dauber:

The Mud Dauber is also a wasp, with a black body, blue luster, and markings around the threaded waist. It is more common to places like Florida.

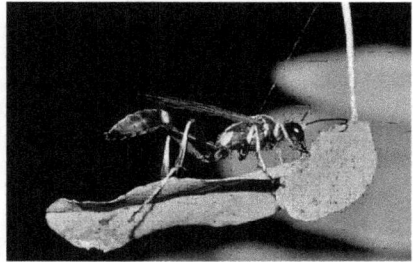

These six bees and wasps are just a few of the species that exist with stingers. They are also the most commonly seen. For example, there is a paper wasp that is less likely to sting a person. It will do so if provoked. The Dirt Dauber, like the Mud Dauber, has a stinger but is only likely to do sting if provoked.

The downside with wasps and bees is you never know what might provoke it to sting. You might be walking by, unaware it is there, and then you have been stung.

Not all bees and wasps will be around flowers. Many will take up residence in the eaves of buildings or outdoor lamps. You do need to check trees for nests, which can be reasonably large when you are outdoors and in the wild. A nest can show several bees or wasps are nearby, and you want to avoid the area.

Chapter 5

Spiders

Types of spiders' number in the thousands. You will want to research where you may be visiting to determine whether there are a considerable number of poisonous spiders in the region. If you have never researched the spiders around your hometown, you may want to do so, to prevent any emergencies with spiders.

As the introduction discussed, sometimes a bite from a small household spider can lead to a large reaction in your body. It all depends on where the bite occurs. Most researchers are going to tell you a spider will not bite unless provoked. You could be sleeping, and the spider bites you. Of course, researchers also say it is more likely an ant that did the deed versus a spider, but if you have noticed spiders in your home or around your camping site, then it may not be an ant at all.

Most people get into trouble with spiders by not recognizing the dangerous insects that are around their home. So, a quick guide into the types of spiders will be provided, and then information on how to deal with the more poisonous bites when they happen will be explained.

It should be noted that not all spiders which look dangerous are poisonous or deadly. Sometimes myths far outweigh the truth. A good example is the camel spider. In 2004, it was purported that the camel spider could be several feet in size, nearly the length of a man's calf or thigh. The scientific community immediately launched their rebuttal of the incident explaining that a camel spider can be at most 4 centimeters in length. The other fact is these spiders are not prone to biting humans, and they do not have the deadly toxins that some of the world's most dangerous spiders have.

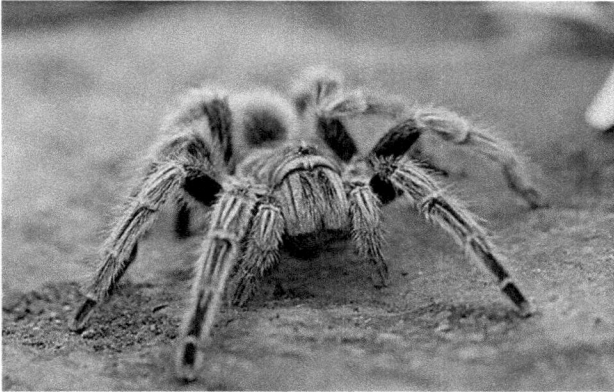

Tarantulas are another fierce creature that is given a bad reputation. Tarantulas are big, hairy spiders, but they do not have a neurotoxin like the brown recluse or black widow. In fact, they rarely bite a human and are kept as pets because they are non-aggressive and not dangerous to humans.

Most of the spiders discussed regarding emergency care are under the tab of "deadly only in extreme cases," meaning a person must have an allergy to the spider venom or be given enough of a dose that it is life-threatening. Most spiders, even the black widow, does not bite with enough envenomation to cause a severe or deadly reaction. The following spiders can be deadly to a select few, some even up to 20% of those they bite, but bites are rare because they are only aggressive when threatened or encountered in a tight space like a shoe, clothing, bedding, or around their eggs.

There are preventative measures to avoiding any spider bite, whether you are out camping, at home, or leasing a space for a holiday.

1. Avoid dark, dry spaces like crawlspaces, basements, garages, woodsheds, woodpiles, and dark, cold vegetative areas.

2. Shake out your clothing, shoes, and bedding before getting into anything, even a sleeping bag.

3. Keep your home sprayed for pests to avoid allowing spiders to nest or lay eggs around your home.

4. If renting, leasing, or staying in a hotel/motel on vacation, double-check the room and bedding. If you spot a spider, ask housekeeping about their pest control methods. Notably, in places like Australia, which is known to have at least two deadly spiders that require antivenom if bitten.

A good rule of thumb when dealing with spiders is to get to a medical facility quickly if you have any concern over the spider being venomous. It is better to be cautious than to realize later that enough envenomation occurred to cause serious harm to you or another person's health.

Each spider will be discussed, but here are a few general treatment considerations:

- Try to kill the spider, if you see it and bring it with you to the medical facility.

- Check to make sure the area is clear of any other potential bites.

- Provide first aid based on the symptoms.

- If a severe reaction occurs, you may need to administer oxygen or CPR to resuscitate the person.

- Hysteria and shock can happen if the person has arachnophobia or if it was one of the more poisonous spiders.

Brown Recluse

The United States is known for its brown recluse spider, although it can live in other regions. The brown recluse can grow to be 6 up to 20 millimeters. However, some have been known to grow much larger. Its name denotes the color, although the back end can be a deep brown or black color to the naked eye. Brown recluse tend to live near woodpiles, sheds, garages, closets, cellars, and other dry, undisturbed spaces. They tend

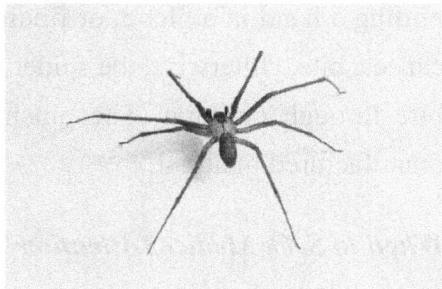

to inhabit cardboard, so if you have any storage boxes and notice spider webs, it is a smart idea to let a bug bomb off before you move those boxes.

Brown recluse bites are usually not felt right away. They may not be painful the first moment you see the bite. However, because they have "hemotoxic" venom, the bite can go from minor to deadly. Hemotoxin destroys red blood cells, which can affect blood clotting, cause skin or tissue damage, and lead to organ degeneration.

A minor bite will appear as a welt, maybe slightly painful, but necrosis will not present. Studies show that 37% of brown recluse bites will cause skin necrosis, while only 14% will show a range of hemotoxic reactions.

The brown recluse is thought to be one of the deadliest spiders in the United States. However, when you look at the statistics, the number of people with allergic reactions is low. This is due to the spider not biting unless provoked, so accidentally sliding a foot in a shoe, putting a hand in a glove, or finding one in the bedsheets will often cause a bite. Otherwise, the spider will leave humans alone. It cannot bite through clothing. The pinchers are too small to go through manufactured material.

When to Seek Medical Attention

The brown recluse bite can still cause a person problems if it occurs. While it may not be life-threatening or even cause necrosis of the skin, you should not ignore the symptoms of a brown recluse bite.

You should seek medical attention if:

- You feel the pain that extends beyond the welt.

- The area becomes swollen.

- You have trouble breathing.

- You notice darkness to your skin.

For example, the welt may be less than a dime in size, but the area of the bite can swell or inflame. Beyond that area, the skin or muscles may feel painful. It can seem like there should be a bruise, but it is swollen and painful instead.

Anytime you have trouble breathing after a suspected insect bite, including a spider bite, you need to visit a doctor to ensure you do not have an apoplectic reaction. It can be mild, but prolonged, you can feel uncomfortable.

Lastly, a dark or black spot around the bite can show necrosis. Sometimes the wound just scabs, and often doctors misdiagnosis a small amount of necrosis. One way to know is to look at the area with a magnifying glass or seek a dermatologist.

The example in the introduction was told the wound just scabbed over; however, there was never an opening to the wound, and the black skin started to appear three days after the bite. Furthermore, the chin wound after the infection of the bite was gone showed a dent where the skin turned black. Thankfully, the doctor did prescribe a topical medicine to help with the skin issue, which prevented further spread and damage, despite just thinking it was a scab.

People who have left necrosis and prolonged swelling from a brown recluse have had significant health problems. They have also lost a significant amount of skin around the wound that remains scarred. It is not something you want to leave.

Now that you understand when to seek medical attention, even if it is several days after a bite, we can look at what to do the minute you realize a brown recluse has bitten you.

Emergency Car for a Brown Recluse Bite

The bite may not itch, even after a few days. It can appear like a massive zit or red welt. If you experience breathing troubles or a change in blood pressure, get to a medical professional immediately, otherwise, follow these instructions.

1. Wash the area.

2. Apply ice to the welt. Ice will help with the inflammation.

3. Feel for any tenderness that may spread around the bite. Your muscles or glands may become swollen if you are having more than a mild reaction to a spider bite.

4. Do not break the skin. Typically, there are small, microscopic holes where the pinchers went in.

5. Apply a topical anti-itch cream or fluid to prevent you from scratching at the welt if you feel an itch.

6. Start Benadryl or a similar medication. Benadryl has diphenhydramine, which is an antihistamine. Any

antihistamine medication can relieve a reaction to insect bites.

7. You want to bandage the bite to ensure you do not scratch it; especially, during sleep.

For a brown recluse, you want to check your symptoms. If the surrounding area of the bite becomes tender, increases in size, or you notice inflammation of the skin, seek medical attention; otherwise, you can continue taking Benadryl to help combat the poison injected by the spider.

- It can take 3 to 8 hours for the area to become inflamed. The skin can appear dry and sinking, bluish, or red near the lesion with a pale center. Typically, the welt resembles a blister. If any of this occurs, seek a doctor, and have your blood count checked for any hemotoxic reaction or infection.

- After 3 to 5 days, the venom is localized to the central area of the bite, and any discomfort will go away.

- However, 7 to 14 days after a bite, you may experience a growing blister or necrosis of the skin.

- It can take up to 3 weeks for the wound to heal, depending on how severe your reaction is.

Black Widow

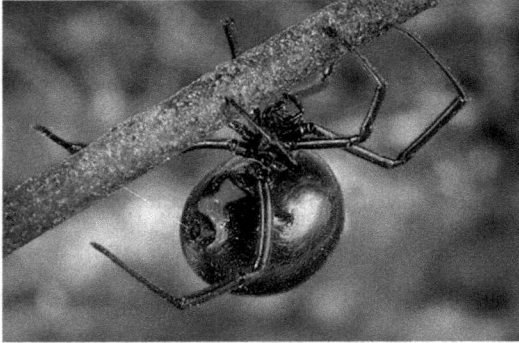

The black widow spider is highly feared because of its venom, and scientists have reported the venom as being ten times stronger than a rattlesnake. Black widow spiders are found in temperate regions. It is a black spider with a red spot on its back. It also has an hourglass shape on the abdomen. The female black widow spider will kill the males after mating. Despite all the bad press these spiders get, they are rarely fatal to humans.

Black widows are found in the US, southern Europe, Africa, Asia, South America, and Australia. They tend to live in the western and southern states of the US. Like the brown recluse, the black widow likes dark, dry locations, such as garages, barns, basements, stumps, rodent holes, brush, trash, dense vegetation, and restrooms.

Also, like brown recluse spiders, the black widow is unlikely to bite unless disturbed. So, the movies that show a black widow crawling over a sleeping person and biting the person who is not moving is not correct. Females are more poisonous than the males and can be considered a threat to human health. Individuals most at risk for a bite from a black widow are young, old, or ill individuals.

A bite will feel like a pinprick or even be unfelt. The pain usually starts within a few moments and will spread to other parts of the body. Nausea, abdominal and back pain, sweating, muscle aches, and hypertension can result. Paralysis of the diaphragm can also lead to breathing issues. However, this does not mean every person reacts the same. This is a more severe reaction. The pain can last for 12 hours, while other symptoms can last for several days.

Those who do not have a reaction to the spider will notice a little localized pain, a rash, and itching, perhaps a little sweating. Those who have a more severe response may not feel their muscles stiffen or hurt until almost 8 hours have gone by after a bite. Depending on the reaction, eyelids can become swollen, and tremors may occur in the legs.

A reaction to a spider bite is also determined by where the spider bites a person. In a fatty area, the bite may not cause the same reactions as being bitten on the face, hands, ankles, feet, or along the spine. Venom can spread, but it will spread quicker in vascular (areas with more blood flow) areas.

Initial Treatment

If breathing or heart troubles present after a bite, seek medical attention immediately, otherwise follow these steps and check your condition.

1. Wash the area where the bite occurred.

2. Use an ice pack to reduce any swelling.

3. Take Benadryl or another antihistamine.

4. Take a pain reliever.

5. Elevate your extremities if the bite occurred on an arm or leg to help with the swelling.

6. Apply an antibiotic cream to the bite.

7. Apply an anti-itch cream if there is itching to avoid scratching the area and opening a wound that could lead to another type of infection.

8. Seek medical attention if the bite becomes worse in looks or you experience extreme pain, paralysis, or tremors.

If you see the spider that bites you and can kill it, do so and bring it to your doctor's appointment. It will help the medical professional confirm the type of spider that bites you.

You need to visit your doctor if you suspect a black widow bite you. They will check the area of the bite, and depending on your symptoms; they can provide antivenom.

If you have an autoimmune disease, compromised health, or are elderly, you should always seek a medical professional after a suspected black widow bite. Any child should be taken quickly to urgent care or emergency room because it can be fatal or extremely detrimental to their health.

Unlike the brown recluse, you can see the puncture wounds of a black widow. The bite of a black widow spider does not, typically, lead to necrosis of the skin. However, you should always be aware that each person will react differently to spider bites.

Banana Spider

The Brazilian wandering spider or banana spider can be aggressive. The wandering spiders are usually found on banana leaves; hence, their other name. You should not confuse this spider with the US banana spider that is called the Golden orb. The Brazilian wandering spider is brown, with a hairy body and long pincers. The banana spider that lives in the southern US states is a Golden orb with a black and yellow appearance. It can be two to three inches in size. The Golden orb is not considered deadly, while the actual banana spider or Brazilian wandering spider can be. This spider does not prefer to bite humans but will when threatened. The bite is usually uncomfortable, but not as harmful as the black widow or brown recluse.

A bite can appear red, with pain around the blister or welt that forms. An allergic reaction can occur, which will include breathing issues, swelling, and hives. Within minutes, an allergic reaction, if there is one, will present with sweating or goosebumps, a change in blood pressure, nausea, vertigo, vision issues, abdominal cramping, and can lead to convulsions.

For men, a prolonged erection can occur due to the boost in nitric oxide, which increases blood flow. According to research by Vetter, 2.3 percent of bites require antivenom, and only 10 deaths can be attributed to the spider in Brazil. This was a study conducted in 2008, and it shows that over time only 10 deaths occurred, not just in one year. Worldwide the number of deaths is approximately 53, after 1980, when the antivenom was created. About 96% of patients will experience severe pain, without respiratory issues or death.

The spider is less likely to use up enough venom to do personal harm, and only about 0.5 percent of cases have severe envenomation that leads to death.

Emergency Care for Banana Spider Bites

If a Brazilian wandering spider truly bites, you seek medical attention. In the wrong place, a bite can block the nervous system and cause death within two hours. It is more likely that mild discomfort will occur. Antivenom is available for any bite by this type of spider.

When you first suspect a banana spider bite, you should do the following:

1. Start driving to an emergency facility.

2. Clean the wound, if possible.

3. Apply ice to the welt that forms to help with inflammation.

4. Ask your physician what types of medication you can take if your symptoms remain mild. A physician may prescribe an antihistamine and pain reliever as the only course of action if a mild reaction occurs. You can buy these over the counter; however, it is advisable to get a doctor's approval for any medication before taking it because they can bring on symptoms related to the spider bite. For example, aspirin can thin the blood and cause heart troubles associated with the toxin in your body.

You want to seek medical care even if you do not feel an allergic reaction or severe envenomation has occurred. Likely, the doctor will look at the bite and send you home to self-monitor your symptoms.

However, you do not want to wait around to see if a delayed reaction will occur.

Due to the low incidents of respiratory failure and death, antivenom is not often used. However, to help counteract any reaction to the venom, a doctor may provide narcotics for pain control or offer an antibiotic to reduce infection.

When venom enters the body, a person's immune system reacts. How severely it reacts will determine how threatening the immune system thinks the substance is. Due to the neurotoxic quality of the venom, patients can suffer dizziness, pain, and tachycardia (increased heart rate), along with vision impairment. With quick treatment, a patient survives the bite.

Yellow Sac Spider

Yellow Sac spiders are 3 to 15 mm in size and tend to live near stones, leaves, and grass. It is named for its color. The entire body is yellow, although the legs can be black at the tips. The spider lives in the lower US, Mexico, and throughout South America. The spider's venom contains cytotoxin, which can destroy cells and impair function, in a high enough dose to humans. Like the brown recluse, it is known to create necrotizing lesions in some people. It is usually found indoors, so it is essential for anyone visiting an area where it is commonly found to be alert.

Despite a rare bite, if one is bitten, the site will generally become red and swell. The female spiders are more aggressive, mainly if they are guarding eggs.

Note: it takes a significant amount of venom to harm a human being. However, if one is particularly susceptible to allergic reactions to insects, it is imperative to seek medical care if bitten by a Yellow Sac spider. Additionally, there are two species under this name, and one is less troubling than the other.

Emergency Care for the Yellow Sac Bite

If bitten, you do want to take proper emergency care, including seeing a medical professional.

1. Wash the area of the bite.

2. Apply ice or a cold washrag to the bite.

3. Monitor yourself or the affected person for an allergic reaction. Some issues may not present until the third day.

4. If there is localized pain, swelling, or shortness of breath, seek medical attention immediately.

5. Before you start taking an allergy medication with antihistamine and a pain reliever, see a medical professional. These medications can mask symptoms the toxin causes or create a more severe medical issue due to the toxin in your body. Never take anything until you have asked a professional.

Your doctor may want to provide an antibiotic to combat the toxin. It will depend on the severity of the symptoms and the area of the bite. Any bite that begins to look necrotic will be attended to with a topical steroid, plus antibiotics.

Always watch a Yellow Sac spider bite for any change in skin color, size, or pain-related symptoms. Get to a doctor if changes occur.

Wolf Spider

The wolf spider is part of a larger group of Lycosidae spiders (Lycosidae is the scientific species name). There is a total of 125 species in North America and about 50 in Europe, as part of this spider species. Due to the many species, there are different looks. However, they tend to be large and hairy, about half-inch to 2 inches in length. They are gray with brown or dark gray markings. Due to the size and color, some people mistake the wolf spider and brown recluse. They do have several characteristics in common with the brown recluse. They like hunting when it is cold and living in dark spaces like basements, closets, and garages.

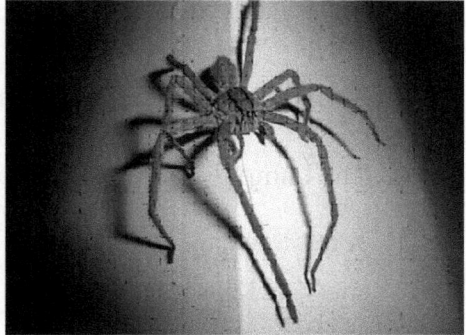

A wolf spider is not aggressive, but if met and threatened may bite. Like most spiders, if you meet it in your bed, it may feel threatened and bite.

While the venom can be harmful to some individuals, a wolf spider is not considered deadly to humans. Most authorities only consider the black widow and brown recluse to be deadly spiders in the US, not wolf spiders.

The bite will typically resemble any other insect bite. You might notice a red welt that is swollen and itchy. Most people find the blister will disappear within a few days without any further trouble. However, an allergic reaction to the venom can occur.

Symptoms of an Allergic Reaction

Specific symptoms mark allergic reactions.

1. The bump increases in size and may resemble hives.

2. A red line can start to extend from the bite area, which would show a blood infection.

3. Breathing issues can present immediately or up to a few hours later.

4. Swelling in the face and around the mouth may present.

5. Extreme reactions include dizziness or a loss of consciousness.

Even with an allergic reaction, a wolf spider bite will not become necrotic or lead to extreme pain and discomfort.

Emergency Care for a Wolf Spider Bite

You will always want to wash the affected area with soap and water.

1. Apply a topical ointment and anti-itch cream to help take the itch out of the bite.

2. Cover the bite with a bandage to prevent scratching. You do not want to create an open wound that could become infected.

3. Take an antihistamine if you have any itching, after speaking with a medical professional and finding out that it is okay.

4. If you or another person experiences shortness of breath, loss of consciousness, or swelling and hives, immediately seek a medical professional.

Brown Widow Spider

Thought to be an African spider, the brown widow can be found in Africa and South America. It is also considered a highly invasive species, having made its way into Southern California, the southern US states, the Caribbean, South Africa, Japan, Australia, Madagascar, and Cyprus. Like most spiders, this species enjoys buildings, old tires, being under automobiles, shrubs, and plants.

The spider ranges from tan to black in color. Some have an ornate brown, black, yellow, white, or orange markings on the abdomen. It is hourglass in shape. Scientists believe the brown widow has a bite that is "twice as powerful" as the black widow, (Britannica, 2020). Like the black widow, the spider is not aggressive and usually wastes a tiny amount of venom when biting a human.

To date, only 2 people in the 1990s have died from a brown widow spider bite. Both individuals suffered from poor health and did not receive antivenom.

The female brown widow has the most venom, and it will inject a neurotoxic venom (a toxin that affects the nervous system) into its prey. Males, according to research, do not bite. The consensus is that the female brown widow spider injects less venom than the Black widow spider, so a reaction may not be as common.

Bites, while uncommon, do happen, and will be shown by a red welt on the skin. Patients usually feel pain, locally, around the wound. For most, the bite is not life-threatening.

If enough toxin is released into the victim, or there is an allergic reaction, it is imperative to seek medical attention.

Symptoms of a Brown Widow Bite

The most common symptoms are:

1. Pain when bitten

2. Red bump near the damaged area

3. Pain or discomfort around the bite

Emergency Care for Brown Widow Bites

You can treat a brown widow bite at home, without seeking medical attention, in most cases. But if any breathing issues arise, heart rate changes or dizziness present seek medical care immediately.

1. Wash the bite with warm, soapy water, and pat the skin dry.

2. Apply ice or a cold cloth to the skin to help reduce swelling around the bite area.

3. If possible, keep the bite elevated to help minimize swelling.

4. Use an anti-itch cream on the bite to help reduce itching.

5. Ask a doctor about over-the-counter medications you can take. You may want to take an antihistamine or pain reliever if you feel prolonged discomfort.

6. You should always seek professional medical assistance if the bite appears to get worse, shows signs of infection or pus is excreted from the wound. If you develop a fever or your skin around the bite becomes warm, you will need to see a doctor.

As always, if an allergic reaction presents later than when the bite occurred, with pain, swelling, and breathing troubles, seek medical help right away. You may be able to reduce the issues with an antihistamine; however, a medical professional may be against this self-administration due to reactions with the toxin. When breathing, loss of consciousness, or extreme pain continues, you need a medical professional.

Red Widow Spider

The red widow spider is characterized by red legs, a black body, with a red head and red markings on the body. Like other "widow" spiders, it has an hourglass shape. Adult females can be 1.5 to 2 inches in length, while the male is a third of that size. The red widow is a Florida native; However, scientists believe it is starting to expand into other parts of the US. It bites when protecting its eggs or if it gets trapped against a person's skin. It has a similar bite to the black widow, with pain, cramping, and nausea. Death is rare due to the small amount of venom injected during a bite. However, elderly, young children and those with health problems are susceptible to increased symptoms and possibly death without treatment.

Treating a Red Widow Spider Bite

If you know a red widow spider bit you or someone else, you will need to keep a careful eye on the symptoms. For most people, a red welt, with localized discomfort is common. However, for those with an allergic reaction or intolerance to low amounts of venom, the following can occur:

- Pain that spreads from the welt

- Inflammation around the wound

- Abdominal cramping

- Nausea

- Trouble breathing

- Muscle pain

Check a patient for any swelling, particularly in the face and around the throat. Any trouble breathing, hives, or significant pain requires a doctor's visit.

Like with the black widow and brown widow, there are antivenoms to help a person combat the effects of the toxin. At the very least, antihistamines, a local anti-itch cream, and potentially, an antibiotic will be necessary to treat the effects of the venom.

1. Determine if severe symptoms are occurring, and if so, get to a medical facility.

2. If the person seems fine, wash the wound area.

3. Apply an anti-itch cream.

4. Cover the spider bite.

5. Monitor symptoms. If prolonged or increased levels of pain, nausea, or respiratory symptoms present a few minutes to hours later, seek medical help.

6. Speak with a doctor before taking over-the-counter medications like an antihistamine or pain reliever. Some medications may cause a reaction with the toxin worsening mild symptoms.

Redback Spider

It is easy to confuse the redback spider with the black widow due to the similarities in their looks and the fact that they are considered "cousin" species. The redback spider is common to Australia but has spread to New Zealand, Japan, and Belgium, through grapes. The spider likes to build webs on grape leaves but does not do well in extremely cold or hot desert conditions. It has a black body, with a red marking on the back. They are not aggressive, and only females bite when disturbed.

Both females and males can bite, but most venomous bites result from the female. About 10 to 20 percent of people bitten experience an envenomation. The neurotoxin will produce swelling in the lymph nodes, an irregular heartbeat, sweating, and pain. According to Britannica, 250 or more redback spider bites are treated in Australia each year, many with antivenom. The last death associated with this spider occurred in 1956 before the antivenom was produced.

A person needs to seek treatment if they believe a redback spider did the biting.

Redback Spider Emergency Care

No matter how far you are from a medical facility, follow these steps.

1. Drive to a medical facility or call for help.

2. Wash the area of the bite.

3. Apply a cold compress to the welt to help reduce swelling.

4. Cover the bite to prevent infection.

5. Elevate the bite area, if possible.

6. Do not massage the bite area.

Monitor the person for any breathing issues, swelling of the lymph nodes, fever, sweating, and extreme pain. If someone is having a severe reaction, do not stop to wash the wound or apply a cold compress. However, consult with a medical professional if you provide an antihistamine and a pain reliever to help the person find comfort.

When breathing troubles and extreme pain present quickly, providing medication to alleviate the symptoms can help the patient survive until you get to a medical treatment facility, where antivenom may be administered. However, some are known to interact negatively with the toxin, so you should ask a doctor before providing anything.

Redback spider antivenom is not available on the market for purchase to keep in your medical kit. It is something you must find at a medical facility.

You should know what this spider looks like, avoid touching grapes (around the leaves), and check your clothing before you put it on to avoid a bite. Given the percentage of potential venomous bites, caution is necessary when visiting or living in Australia.

Funnel-Web Spider

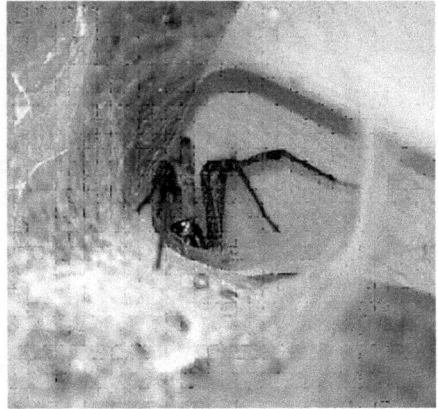

The funnel-web spider is named for the web they spin. It is a more massive spider with hairy legs and a black and brown body, mostly a dark color with lighter rings on the legs and stripes on the face. The funnel-web spider has several species, three that live in the US, one in South America, and one in Australia. However, not all Funnel-web spiders are considered poisonous. The Atrax genus, living in Australia, is the poisonous spider. It is highly feared in the southern and eastern parts of Australia. Death has occurred from these Australian species. Studies started recording deaths in the 1920s. According to the Australian Museum, only 13 deaths have occurred from funnel-web spiders in Australia. The Guardian, a UK newspaper, lists 14 reported deaths and states death can occur in 15 minutes. The spiders are considered aggressive.

An antivenom must be provided as soon as a victim has been bitten to prevent death or severe impairment. The antidote takes care of the main toxin injected during a bite.

A person should consider any funnel-web spider bite by the Australian Atrax to be medically dangerous. Paralysis at the site of the bite or orally can occur. Muscle spasms, abdominal pain, vomiting, headache, nausea, pulmonary edema, myocardial (heart troubles) injury and central nervous effects such as anxiety, drowsiness, or coma can occur in severe bites.

Emergency Care for the Funnel Web Spider Bite

If you suspect a funnel-web spider has bitten you:

1. Get in a vehicle immediately.
2. Drive to the nearest medical facility.

Whether you are by yourself or helping someone, you need to get medical attention. Antivenom can be the difference between life and death.

Check with a medical professional as you or another person may be able to take an antihistamine to counteract an allergic reaction. It may also help you or the patient while you wait for medical attention and antivenom.

- If traveling to Australia, always bring an antihistamine with you and carry it with you.

- For those living in Australia, an antihistamine should be a part of every emergency medical kit.

An antihistamine is designed to reduce allergies, including any trouble with a restricted airway. It will not prevent the toxin from spreading or prevent death. However, it can help you remain capable of breathing until you reach a medical facility, providing you do not have an adverse reaction to the antihistamine and toxin being in your system together.

Taking a pain reliever can also help reduce the pain you experience in your muscles. Still, aspirin is a blood thinner, so any signs of heart troubles mean you should not take a pain reliever, even acetaminophen (Tylenol).

Toxin from spiders is known to cause an irregular heartbeat. Aspirin is a known helper for those suffering from a heart attack because it helps increase blood flow. However, a toxin from a spider bite can cause red blood cells to burst and cause hemolysis. There is no clear medical description for whether aspirin should be administered to help regulate the heart and blood flow when injected with funnel-web spider venom. Aspirin is also designed to lower high blood pressure, so if you are experiencing low blood pressure due to a spider bite, it is not a promising idea to take aspirin.

1. During the drive, immobilize the bite area, such as an arm or leg, but do not abnormally restrict blood flow to the area. You want to reduce the spread of the toxin, without endangering the area of the bite.

2. Apply a cold compress to the area to help reduce swelling.

Allergic reactions to funnel-web spider bites are rare. Current treatment says a patient should apply the pressure bandage and get to the hospital. Medical professionals will administer the antivenom in two vial. This can be repeated every 15 to 30 minutes until any envenoming issue is resolved. Patients are also seen for 2 to 4 hours after a bite. Only once the antivenom is available should the pressure bandage be removed. If it appears there is no severe envenoming after 4 hours, a patient may be able to go home.

However, all large brown spider bites in Australia should be treated as a funnel-web spider bite, even though a mouse spider bite is similar in appearance. Furthermore, some people do not immediately show envenomation symptoms, which is why a person needs to be checked, even at home, after a suspected funnel-web spider bite. Always seek immediate medical care if symptoms worsen.

Hobo Spider

The hobo spider is part of the genus that belongs to the funnel-web spider; however, it is not like the Australian funnel-web spider. The Centers for Disease Control and Prevention (CDC) does not consider the hobo spider to have any toxic effects on humans. The hobo spider is found in the Pacific Northwest of the United States in places like Washington, Oregon, Utah, and Idaho. The common name of the spider came from finding it along railroad tracks. But it also likes holes, cracks, rock, construction supplies, and foundations.

The hobo spider does not like to live in houses. It is a brown spider with long legs and a black and tan body, although sometimes it is noted to have yellow markings. The spider is usually a quarter to a half-inch in length and has 1 to 2 inches of leg.

Most hobo spider bites occur in the summer months when the females are searching for males. People do not usually feel the bite or might feel like a pinpricked them. In 2014, Oregon medical staff did verify an allergic reaction to a hobo spider bite by an individual. The person had redness, pain, and leg twitching for 12 hours. However, after necrosis set in, the team and the Centers for Disease Control and Prevention changed their mind. The hobo spider is not known to cause any necrosis, even if there is an allergic reaction.

If you are bitten by a spider and can catch or kill it, you should. If you experience any allergic reaction or suspected toxicity, take the spider to a medical facility to help the staff verify the bite and the culprit.

Since hobo spider bites are not considered toxic to humans, the treatment is simple.

Treatment for a Hobo Spider Bite
As always, monitor you or the person bitten for an allergic reaction and seek medical help if one presents.

1. Clean the area of the bite with soap and warm water.

2. Apply a cold compress to the area of the bite to help reduce any swelling or pain.

3. Elevate the area where the bite occurred, if possible.

4. Use an anti-itch cream to prevent scratching.

You should also consider taking an antihistamine for a day or two if there is extended pain near the bite site or added swelling. While an allergic reaction or toxicity is unfounded from a hobo spider bite, you do want to be cautious and monitor the bite. Any change in your health could mean an allergic reaction or that you were incorrect in identifying the spider.

Spiders and Toxicity

There are very few "deadly" spiders in the world. While they are deadly to small insects or rodents, the toxicity level in a bite is typically low enough to avoid killing a human. As you read above, there are a few exceptions like the funnel-web spider.

You never want to avoid seeking proper medical attention from a spider bite if you experience severe symptoms. It can mean you were wrong about the type of spider, or you may have an unnatural intolerance to a spider's venom. A simple bite on the face can also be cause for alarm because of the vascular nature of the skin. It is easier to obtain a higher level of venom in your blood from a bite on the face than in other areas of the body.

You can also develop a blood condition if an infection sets in, so when a doctor or nurse practitioner sees an allergic reaction to a spider bite, they will often run a CBC panel to check your blood cell counts. If there is a change in the level that suggests infection, they may need to prescribe medication. Furthermore, if it has been 10 years since your last tetanus shot, they will probably provide a booster shot to help stave off any infection.

You want to be incredibly careful when obtaining medications for spider bites. The ideal choice is an antibiotic; however, it may not be penicillin or derivatives of the first antibiotic. It could have a sulfonamide. Sulfa antibiotics like Bactrim have a similar component to shellfish. A person can develop a skin rash, itching, headache, dizziness, diarrhea, tiredness, nausea, vomiting, pale skin, joint pain, and sensitivity to light due to an allergic reaction to the antibiotic.

The worst part about antibiotics—if you have never had the one prescribed—you can go the full 14-day treatment without appearing allergic to it.

You want to keep track of any allergies to antibiotics, medications, and spiders to help medical professionals treat you accordingly. Furthermore, what you do in the field can help save a life if there is an allergic reaction.

Chapter 6

Scorpions

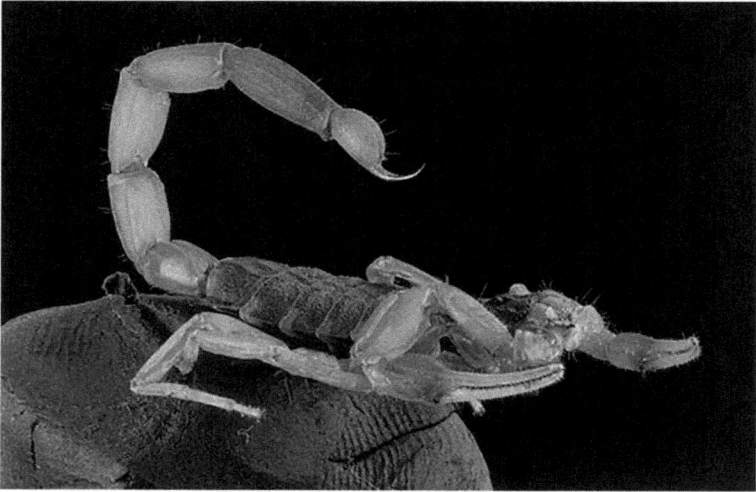

Plenty of "deadly" insects exist, from ants to scorpions if you are a small rodent, insect, young, elderly, or ill person. This section will examine scorpions and their toxicity levels. Like spiders, it takes a significant amount of toxin for many of these scorpions to lead to death. However, some will undoubtedly kill and others that can cause an allergic reaction that can be lethal. Infection can also set in, which is not a result of the insect but rather the care of the bite area.

There are several types of scorpions. They dwell in desert and warm climates like Arizona, Africa, the Middle East, Asia, and even Florida. They spend their days in holes, rocks, or burrows, hiding from the sun. At night scorpions will come out to hunt small rodents like mice, opossums, rats. They also kill birds and centipedes.

Most scorpions will be on the level of a bee sting, irritating, slightly painful, but otherwise not harmful to humans. It is said a baby scorpion can have a higher rate of envenomation, depending on the species. Some species contain a neurotoxin that can be deadly to humans. The toxin affects the central nervous system paralyzing the victim, including making it impossible to breathe. The deathstalker scorpion is said to be one of the deadliest, even to humans. Despite these scorpions and others causing death, the same rules apply as those with spiders—young, elderly, or infirm—are most susceptible. A healthy person can usually survive toxic scorpions. You do not want to find out, and if stung, you do need to seek medical attention.

You will want to bring the scorpion with you for identification purposes if you can. It is possible to be stung by a nonlethal scorpion, so knowing which species did the deed is imperative to proper medical care.

According to Mayo Clinic researchers, only 30 scorpion species of 1500 can produce a toxic venom that would prove fatal to humans. National Geographic states there are 2,000 species of scorpions, and 30 to 40 of them have enough venom to kill a person. The 7 deadliest scorpions are overviewed here, with treatment for stings. Over a million scorpion stings occur each year, with a moderate amount of deaths, which is why understanding the medical care required is imperative.

Bark Scorpion

American Survival Guide Magazine wrote a piece about the bark scorpion given its prevalence in North America. It is found in Arizona, New Mexico, Nevada, Utah, and Mexico. The study showed that venom does contain a potent neurotoxin that will cause pain for its subject. Patients have stated it is like getting an electrical jolt. Severe cases have led to numbness, vomiting, and diarrhea. The symptoms, if severe enough, can lead to death due to dehydration and anaphylaxis. If the bark scorpion sting is left untreated, it can lower one's rate of survival by 1 to 25% based on the victim's health and age. There is an antivenom. The last known death from a bark scorpion sting in the US was 40 years ago.

The bark scorpion is slender, with a thin tail and thin pincers compared to other scorpions. It is tan or yellowish-brown in color. It can also have markings or stripes that go from head to tail. The Sonora (a type of bark scorpion) is different because it has an entirely black body, with a yellow tail, legs pincers, and stinger. There is also a triangle on its head. The bark scorpion is about 2.75 to 3 inches for both females and males, respectively.

For emergency care:

1. Wash the area of the sting.

2. Monitor your health.

3. Cover the welt with a cold compress or ice.

4. Seek a medical facility as soon as possible.

5. Take a pain reliever, such as acetaminophen (Tylenol). You should not take aspirin or ibuprofen as both could contribute to neuro issues.

6. Do not cut the wound or apply suction.

7. You cannot apply a tourniquet around the sting area.

8. Do immobilize the sting area.

A tourniquet at the correct pressure can help prevent the toxin flowing too fast but is not considered adequate or proper medical care. You never want to open the wound or use suction to try to get the venom out, as this can lead to infection and a more troubling recovery than the sting itself.

When you visit a medical facility, they will likely provide antibiotics only if they are worried about the infection of the sting area or if your blood cell counts indicate an infection is occurring. Antibiotics do not help reduce or stop the effects of the venom.

You should always seek a medical professional if a child, elderly person, or ill person has been stung. If you are out in the desert and hours from any medical facility, you can call for the emergency department to send out help with antivenom. Due to the prohibitive cost of producing the approved antivenom, it is not available for purchase, privately.

Deathstalker Scorpion

If you live in the US and never plan to visit the Middle East and North Africa, then you will be safe from the deathstalker scorpion. It is native to the desert countries like Algeria, Chad, Egypt, Israel, Ethiopia, Jordan, and Somalia.

Unlike the scorpions in the movie, this one is translucent yellow with a slightly dark back. The color can vary between yellow and orange-brown.

Clinical evidence suggests the deathstalker scorpion has a deadly neurotoxin, but it doesn't have some of the other venoms like myotoxin, procoagulant, anticoagulant, hemorrhagin, nephrotoxin, cardiotoxin, or necrotoxin. However, it is still an uncomfortable venom since it targets the nervous system. It will not cause hemorrhages or necrosis of the skin.

The information states it has a dangerous level of envenoming that can be lethal. The rate of envenoming is 80%, which means it provides a dose of venom in 80% of stinging cases, with an untreated lethality rate of 1 to 10%. This means only 1 to 10 percent of people stung who leave the condition untreated die from the envenomation.

The effects around the sting area include pain and swelling. No cases of necrosis have been seen, according to CDC and other reporting agencies. However, there can be systemic effects or symptoms like headache, abdominal pain, nausea, diarrhea, respiratory distress, dizziness, hypotension, convulsions, or collapse.

If you suspect someone or you have encountered a deathstalker scorpion and been stung, you need to make sure there is no further risk of stings. Make sure the area is clear and attempt to kill the scorpion without further injury to you or anyone else.

1. Have the person lie down. It is essential to become prone and still. Due to the pain and fear of scorpion death, patients can irrationally react or become hysterical. Even with the deathstalker, death is rare.

2. The sting wound should not be touched, except with a cool cloth to clean the area quickly.

3. Do not massage the wound, cut it open, or attempt to suction out the venom.

4. A cold compress has been considered helpful to alleviate pain around the wound, but there is no clinical proof of this.

5. Due to inflammation, if the wound is on the arm or hand, the jewelry should be removed.

6. The stung area needs to be immobilized, with a temporary splint or sling. A tourniquet is not something that should be used. While it may seem essential to cut off the blood supply and stop the venom from spreading, a tourniquet has shown to do more harm than good for the person stung.

7. Any respiration or airway troubles should be treated with mouth to mouth (mask) to help maintain oxygen flow for the individual. If you have an oxygen tank with a mask, that is the best option. The venom can damage heart function and

circulation, and CPR may be required. (Refer to section 1 for CPR instructions).

The bite area must remain immobile. Moving an affected limb, such as walking to an emergency location, can cause the venom to spread. The patient should be strapped to a stretcher and carried out, carried on some-one's back, or otherwise remain immobile until treatment can be provided.

If at all possible, bring the dead scorpion with you to the emergency facility.

Alcohol or sedatives should not be given to the patient. Only a qualified medical person should prescribe medications. In many instances, antivenom is required to help a person stung by a deathstalker scorpion.

Clinically, no folk or traditional remedy outside of correct medical care has shown effectiveness against a deathstalker scorpion sting. Even using a "venom apparatus" has not been proven to work. The wound should not be excised or otherwise touched as this could cause infection rather than help the individual survive the bite.

Spitting Thick-Tail Black Scorpion

The Spitting Thick-tail Black scorpion is found in South Africa and is also known as the fat-tail scorpion. It is considered the most dangerous scorpion in the southern regions of the African continent. It has a large tail with a stinger that can release 4.25 milligrams of venom into its prey. According to American Survival Guide Magazine, the 4.25 mg of venom is enough to kill a human. The

WCH Clinical website that provides toxicology information states that this scorpion has an excitatory neurotoxin that can lead to severe envenoming. It can be potentially lethal due to paralysis of the nervous system. However, general clinical effects state the rate of envenoming is less than 80%, and the untreated lethality rate is below 1%.

The American Survival Guide Magazine says the Fat-tail is known to deliver two doses of venom, and it is more likely the second delivery that will cause a fatal envenomation in humans. The reason this scorpion is known as a "spitting" Thick-tail Black scorpion is its color and ability to "spit" its venom. Small targets can become temporarily blind when the venom is "spit" up to three feet.

The low mortality rate for humans stung by this scorpion does not mean a sting is pleasant. Symptoms include:

- Muscular convulsions

- Sweating

- Intense pain

- Heart palpitations

- Drooling

The scorpion is identified by its black color. It can be six inches in size. It has small pincers and a large black tail that can stab its victim and release its venom. It does have hair on its body, which it uses to read the vibrations and disturbances in the air that movement can cause.

Unlike some scorpions, it has a warning sound similar to the rattlesnake because it will rub its stinger across the rough area of its back. While predominately a South African scorpion, it has been seen in the Middle East and other parts of Africa. It prefers a semi-arid location.

You will want to keep away from caves, rocks, crannies, or cacti as it likes to stay in dark, cool places. It hunts at night.

You must understand the proper medical care if you intend to visit or live in a region where it is found.

Emergency Care for the Fat-Tail Spitting Black Scorpion

Make sure the area is clear of the scorpion and any other scorpions. A second sting will almost certainly be lethal if medical attention is not close. Kill the scorpion if it is not dangerous to do so.

1. Attempt to calm the stung person down. All too often, someone stung by a scorpion will panic or become hysterical due to the myths of deadly scorpion stings. The more a person moves, the more the venom has a chance to spread to other parts of the body.

2. The pain is often intense, but you should not attempt to cut or excise the wound in any way, including attempting to suck out the venom.

3. You can clean the area of the sting and cover it to keep it clean.

4. If you have ice or an ice pack, you may try to help the swelling in the area of the sting, but it has not been clinically proven to help in any other way.

5. Depending on the area of the sting, you may need to remove jewelry or shoes in case swelling occurs.

6. Most stings are to a limb, such as a leg or an arm. Immobilize the person, particularly the affected area by using a splint or stretcher.

7. Administer CPR if any impairment occurs to the airway or circulation. Otherwise, keep the person immobile and head to the nearest medical facility you can find.

8. You should not use a tourniquet to try to stop the spread of venom. This will cut off circulation and could do irreparable damage to a person's limb.

9. No alcohol or sedative should be administered as this could cause more health issues or cover those being caused by the venom.

10. Keep the person hydrated; especially, if it will take a long time to reach a medical facility.

Do not cut or cauterize the wound. Do not attempt to use folk or local remedies for envenomation. It is imperative to get a patient to a medical facility as soon as possible. With the fat-tail scorpion, it is not likely antivenom will need to be administered. Still, allergic reactions to the venom need to be monitored, or prolonged symptoms may need more medical treatment. However, for most people, the effects of a fat-tail scorpion bite are short-lived, meaning there are no systemic effects in the majority of humans stung by this scorpion. There is an antivenom called SAIMR produced by South African Vaccine Producers LTD. It is only available at local medical facilities and not available for private purchase.

According to WCH Clinical Toxicology, most fat-tail scorpion stings do not lead to admission, for a prolonged period, at a medical facility. This is due to the two-sting approach. A person is usually alerted to the presence of the scorpion by the first non-lethal sting and able to avoid the second sting that contains a higher dose of antivenom.

You should never consider any scorpion sting as minor until the symptoms indicate only local pain and swelling occur, rather than assuming it is minor and waiting too long to get treatment should a reaction occur.

Yellow Fat-Tail Scorpion

Like the spitting fat-tail black scorpion, the yellow one is named for its color. Its scientific name is "Androctonus" means "man killer" in Greek. It has one of the most potent neurotoxins that any scorpion has. The venom is designed to attack the central nervous system and cause paralysis and respiratory failure in its prey.

The pincers on the yellow fat-tail are small along with the body in comparison to other scorpions; however, its tail is large. The legs, tail, and pincers have yellow, while the body is usually brown or black. It grows to 2.5 up to 3.5 inches in length. This scorpion lives in northern Africa and Southeast Asia.

According to scientific studies, the amount of venom released during a sting is 2.95 milligrams. It is thought to have a neurotoxin and possibly a cardiotoxin. If encountered by a human, it is possible that severe envenoming can occur, with a potentially lethal dose of venom. The envenoming rate is 10 to 20 percent, with an untreated lethality rate between 1 and 10 percent.

In general, a patient will feel:

- Severe pain in the sting area.

- See local redness and sweat.

Systemic effects can occur in a higher envenomation situation:

- Nausea

- Headache

- Vomiting

- Diarrhea

- Abdominal pain

- Respiratory distress

- Dizziness

- Hypotension

- Convulsions or collapse can occur

It is highly unlikely that a sting will cause hemorrhaging or coagulation issues. However, in rare cases, it has been seen as a secondary effect. With severe envenoming, cardiac failure or arrhythmias can occur. Hypovolemic hypotension, which is to say blood pressure issues, can occur due to a high loss of fluid due to sweating and vomiting.

The yellow fat-tail scorpion sting is not pleasant. First, aid should be administered based on the thought of severe envenoming.

Young children, elderly, or at-risk people are more susceptible to severe envenoming. They should not delay in obtaining proper care.

Emergency Care for Yellow Fat-tail

If you suspect or know you or someone in your party has been stung by a yellow fat-tail scorpion, seek the nearest medical facility.

1. Check the area for the scorpion to prevent another sting, as well as any other scorpions that could sting.

2. Attempt to keep the patient calm to prevent further spread of the venom.

3. Immobilize the person or extremity that has sustained the sting.

4. Do not massage, excise, or attempt to remove the venom in any way from the wound.

5. Wash the wound and cover it.

6. You may try to use a cold compress to keep the swelling down, but this is secondary to other medical care.

7. Monitor the patient for any systemic signs, including trouble breathing, a change in blood pressure, or paralysis.

8. Do not provide any medication that could hinder the overall display of symptoms unless it will help open the airway. Scorpion stings can lead to a closed airway, so administering oxygen is helpful.

Administering an antihistamine is not going to help. It is not the closure of the airway from an allergic reaction, but a paralysis of the central nervous system that prevents the brain and body from continuing to keep a person breathing.

9. Get the patient to a medical clinic to obtain antivenom; primarily, if cardio or respiratory distress occurs.

It is essential to know which regions will have the antivenom. In some regions, it is rarely used or avoided altogether due to controversy over its effectiveness. If you are visiting an area that does not believe in antivenom, you may need to request temporary medical care. Alternatively, change your plans and go to a region that will have the Monovalent or anti-scorpionique treatment. Algeria is one region that will use antivenom in treating a patient.

Brazilian Yellow Scorpion

The Brazilian yellow scorpion has a yellowish-brown body, with its legs, tail, and pincers having a pale-yellow appearance. As its name suggests, it is found in Brazil, but also most of South America. It grows up to 2.7 inches. It eats insects and small rodents. It prefers hiding in debris, such as piles of wood by houses.

People are stung each year by this scorpion due to its prevalence in South America. Most of the cases are mild, with the patient feeling pain, fever, sweating, rapid heartbeat, and nausea. However, in more severe instances, a patient can experience hyperesthesia, which means the body becomes paralyzed. In contrast, the patient feels intense pain, stomach cramps, and breathing issues. For the elderly, young, or at-risk person, a Brazilian yellow scorpion sting can lead to death. According to the American Survival Guide Magazine, an average of 3,000 people die from its sting each year despite antivenom protocols. In 2016, the antivenom was listed as not 100% effective. In fact, some people have a lethal allergic reaction to the antivenom.

The venom is considered a neurotoxin and cardiotoxin. Severe envenoming is possible from one sting. Most stings will lead to a local reaction around the wound; however, in children under 14 years of age, it has a 1 percent lethality rate when left untreated. For all other stings, it is under .28%.

Symptoms can include:

- Local swelling and pain around the sting wound.

- Vomiting

- Tachycardia (a rapid heartbeat)

- Sweating

- Restlessness

- Somnolence (sleepiness)

- Hyper or hypothermia

- Hypertension

- Cardiotoxicity with tachycardia

- Less commonly bradycardia, hypertension, and cardiac arrhythmias.

In some patients, a sting has led to heart failure and cardiac arrest, typically in less than 5% of children's cases.

Medical Management for Brazilian Yellow Scorpion Sting

For adults, due to body size, a sting rarely causes a significant dose of envenoming; however, symptomatic care is necessary. Admission to a medical facility may not be required; however, any child under 14 years of age, elderly, or at-risk person should immediately seek medical care. Brazil is known for providing an IV of antivenom in all pediatric cases when a Brazilian yellow scorpion is a culprit.

1. Begin with checking the scorpion is gone or dead, and that no other threat is present.

2. Attempt to calm the patient, as more movement can lead to the spread of the venom. Due to the pain, children can become extremely hysterical or irrational.

3. Depending on the age of the patient, you may decide to wash the wound and immobilize the area. However, for at-risk patients, it is best to start driving to an emergency care facility.

4. If swelling occurs, remove footwear or jewelry that could compromise circulation.

5. Provide CPR if any breathing or heart issues present.

6. Do not try to treat this type of scorpion sting at home.

It is better to seek a medical professional after any scorpion sting, even if your symptoms appear minor. You may need something for the extreme pain the venom can cause or be released to go home. For children, anesthesia, intubation, and ventilation may be necessary to help keep oxygen flow going, as well as to minimize the pain felt by the venom. Kids may be administered beta-blockers or atropine to help with hypertension and circulatory shock.

The Brazilian yellow scorpion lives in highly populated areas and has a severe enough amount of venom that when it stings a human it can lead to death, particularly, in children. You should never ignore the incident.

Arabian Fat-Tailed Scorpion

Many of the most dangerous scorpions have an enormous tail and stinger, which allows them to provide a higher dose of venom into their prey. This makes it particularly dangerous for humans. The Arabian fat-tailed scorpion, like its other species relations, is highly prevalent in Africa and the Middle East. For soldiers serving overseas in the Persian Gulf, these scorpions were considered a significant hazard. Several pop culture references tend to involve the Arabian fat-tailed scorpion.

Turkey has farmed this scorpion for its venom to produce antivenom since 1942. It should be noted the pincers on this scorpion are more significant than other fat-tailed scorpions. This is the black scorpion you see in movies, with the armored exoskeleton, large pincers, and thick curving tail. It can grow up to 4 inches in size. Unlike most of the scorpions discussed above, the Arabian fat-tailed scorpion is aggressive, and it will attack instead of running away if it feels threatened.

It lives in the sand during the day, making it possible to encounter it just by walking along a desert path. It will also hide in ruins, woodpiles, stones, rubble, and in houses. Anything dark and small will attract this scorpion.

This scorpion has an excitatory neurotoxin but does not contain other toxins. Although clinically, it has not been proven to contain cardiotoxins, it has not been ruled out, either. Severe envenoming is possible, with a potentially lethal dose of venom. The envenoming rate is 1o to 20 percent, with an untreated lethality rate of 1 to 10 percent.

For most stings, severe pain, redness, and sweating, limited to the sting area, will occur. It is possible to have systemic effects, including a headache, vomiting, abdominal pain, diarrhea, nausea, respiratory distress, collapse, dizziness, convulsions, or hypotension.

Cardiotoxicity is considered either direct or indirect due to severe envenoming and has led to cardiac failure in some patients. Due to fluid loss, a change in blood pressure has been known to occur.

Emergency Care for an Arabian Scorpion Sting

Always begin by making sure no one is in any more danger of being stung by a scorpion. If at all possible, kill the scorpion, then bring it with you to the emergency facility.

1. Due to the envenomation, this scorpion can lead to; you are better off starting by calming down the patient.

2. Get the person immobile to avoid spreading the venom further in the body. Get the person on a stretcher, laying down in a vehicle, or on their back.

3. Walk or drive to the nearest facility, depending on what you have available unless you can get help to you quicker than you can get to help.

4. Only stop if you need to administer CPR. This scorpion can lead to respiratory and cardiac problems. If vital functions are impaired, attempt to make it easier for the person to breathe or restart their heart. Otherwise, continue to the medical center.

5. Do not avoid seeking professional help.

The Arabian fat-tailed Scorpion envenomation can cause delayed reactions in some patients, meaning the onset of symptoms is not readily apparent. Sometimes the systemic symptoms can appear quickly. You never want to wait even if you or the other person feels no effects.

If a sting leads to local pain, the medical facility may provide anesthetic infiltration at the wound site. However, if more severe symptoms occur, a patient will be admitted, and depending on the region, and antivenom will be used to treat the severe case. Often replacement fluids are provided for sweating and vomiting to prevent dehydration.

When it will take you several hours to get to a medical facility, make sure you help hydrate the person stung.

Medical facilities state: All cases need to be treated as urgent and potentially lethal. You will need to think along these same lines and do what you can to help the patient reach a medical location. However, you should never mess with the wound, attempt to suck out the venom, or stimulate the muscle around the sting as this will lead to more issues.

Indian Red Scorpion

The last scorpion to discuss is the Indian red scorpion. This does not mean other scorpions cannot sting and cause envenomation. Quite the opposite, all scorpions have stingers and, when provoked, can envenom a human. However, the dose of venom dispensed by other species of scorpions has not proven to be lethal, except in rare cases, in the elderly, infirm, or young. Stings are usually painful but not deadly. The Indian red scorpion has a high potential of being lethal.

The Indian red scorpion dwells in India, Pakistan, and several west Asian countries. Its name is derived from the reddish-brown color of its body and tail. However, it can also be yellow or deep brown and its eyes and markings can be black. It is a night hunter of insects, lizards, and mice. It can grow up to 4 inches in size. According to WCH Toxicology, the estimated venom dose is 3.6 milligrams, which, as we saw with other scorpions, is enough to be lethal to a human.

The effects of this scorpion are not as documented as other deadly scorpions. In fact, the WCH does not have any clinical effects or a list of the typical type of venom provided by this scorpion. However, likely, severe pain, vomiting, nausea, dizziness, circulatory, and respiratory issues can present in a high envenoming situation. One source, Planet Deadly, states it is possible to have fluid in the lungs, and cardiac issues result from the toxic venom, and this usually happens to a human within 24 hours.

Seeking immediate medical treatment is necessary. It should be mentioned that most regions where this scorpion is found will not have antivenom procedures. You might be lucky in the larger Indian cities to find antivenom. However, in the smaller locales, the treatment will be to attempt to provide fluids, pain relievers, and treat the symptoms with medication rather than an antivenom.

You can help anyone stung by this scorpion by offering quick medical assistance.

1. Make sure no one is in any more danger of being stung.

2. Kill the scorpion, if at all possible, and bring it to the nearest medical facility for identification.

3. Calm the patient down as best as you can.

4. Immobilize the person, mainly around the wound area, especially if it is a limb. You want to prevent the further spread of venom.

5. Avoid any excising of the wound, suction of the venom, or muscle stimuli as this can lead to more complications.

6. If impairment to vital functions presents, provide CPR.

It is most helpful to carry some type of oxygen with you in your emergency medical kit to help you supply oxygen; especially, if you need to get the heart started again.

Do not provide any medications on site. While pain relievers can help with the excruciating pain, it can mask other symptoms or cause the heart to react erratically.

Your best defense is to get to the nearest medical assistance as quickly as possible.

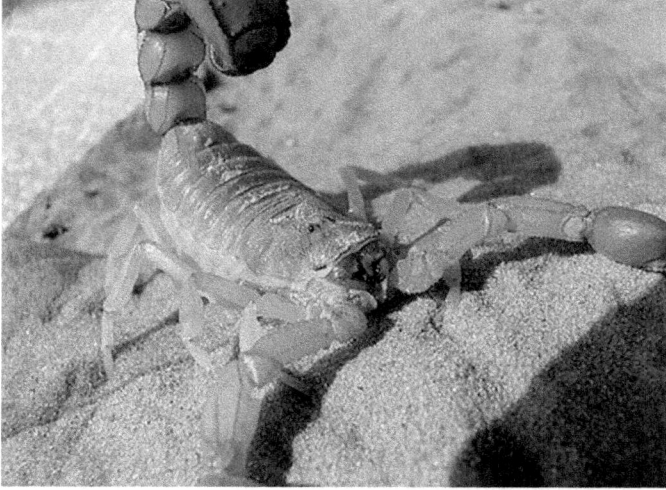

Chapter 7

Ants – Are They Harmful?

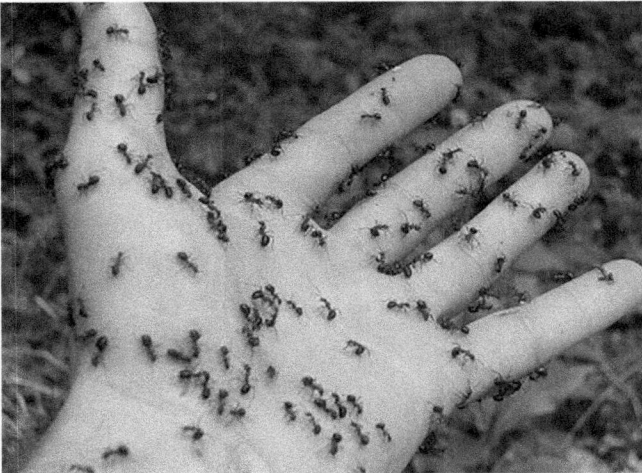

A nts seem harmless enough. They come into our homes, crawl over things, but don't seem to do any harm. But there are always exceptions to the rules. For example, carpenter ants are about a half-inch in length, and they will eat wood. They can "bite," which is more irritating than deadly. Fire ants and red ants are certainly not fun to be around, but again most of the time, they are more irritating than harmful.

Although ant bites are rarely deadly, an allergic reaction or infection at the wound site can lead to death. Ant venom is made by the gastor gland. It is typically a pheromone (hormone scent) communication to tell other ants there is something to eat. The Maricopa harvester ant is considered the most venomous. In contrast, the Bullet ant has the most painful sting on the Schmidt Pain index.

The Maricopa harvester ant is just one type of harvester ant. These ants are known for their larger mandibles that will grind seed into "bread" for storage in their granaries or use in their nests. This ant lives mostly in Southwest America but can be found in Mexico. They live in the desert, with nests that reach 4.5 meters deep. The colony is about 10 thousand ants. While not aggressive, if threatened, the Maricopa will bite or sting, leaving a person feeling a local pain for up to 8 hours. Most people find their sting on the same pain level as a bee.

The Maricopa is just one of 12,500 ant species, according to Lake Norman Pest Control. You should always know what ants are in your area or the place you are going to visit. Make sure you know what they look like and avoid colonies.

The following is going to look at distinct ant species that can cause serious harm to humans and discuss the best emergency care options.

Bulldog Ant

According to the Guinness World Records, the Bulldog Ant (Myrmecia Pyriformis), is the most dangerous ant in the world, and it lives in Australia. Found along the coast, it will sting and bite at the same time. Since 1936, three human deaths have been linked to this ant, including a farmer in 1988.

Due to the aggressive nature of this ant, it is feared. It will bite and sting in quick succession, providing more venom with each sting. The recorded deaths show that an adult died within 15 minutes due to the extreme envenomation. The ant's body length is only 20 millimeters. Thankfully, the lifespan of these ants is 21 days, except for the queen, which can live longer.

Death occurs in those who have allergic reactions to the venom, much like death by a bee. This ant is usually outdoors in soil, under logs, or rocks. It is best to stay away from a colony. If a colony is spotted, proper eradication is necessary.

Care from a Sting

1. Kill the ant immediately. It will continue to bite and sting unless you squash it quickly.

2. Monitor the person, bitten, and stung for any signs of anaphylactic shock, which means breathing issues.

3. Seek medical attention if an allergic reaction occurs—do not let the reaction go untreated.

4. Use an antihistamine to help with the allergic reaction, especially if medical attention is quite a distance from your location. You do not want to provide a pain reliever or antihistamine if it is known to cause erratic heartbeats, as the venom can also increase or decrease heart rate.

Call a medical facility to get appropriate medical advice based on the reaction a person is having to this ant. If you are close enough to a medical facility that can send out an emergency unit, treat the allergic reaction as best you can while you wait for emergency personnel.

If no allergic reaction is seen:

- Clean the bite and sting area with warm soapy water.

- Use a cold compress to help with the local swelling.

- Apply an anti-itch product to help with the itching.

- Cover the wound area to prevent an open sore from occurring.

- Monitor any pain that seems to spread from the wound site.

- If breathing troubles present, seek immediate medical attention.

- Provide a pain reliever if the pain is uncomfortable.

- Monitor the patient for any delayed reaction to the bite.

Death occurs due to restricted airways, so if you can help a person obtain oxygen and get treatment, death is unlikely to occur.

It should also be mentioned: more than one ant, with multiple bites, can lead to severe envenomation and the potential to be lethal. Do not stand around if one ant begins its aggressive attack. Walk away from the area, attempt to kill the ant, and seek medical care. You may not know if you have walked into a colony as they have extensive underground networks.

Siafu Ant

The Siafu ant is an army ant, which lives in Eastern and Central Africa. The Siafu is known to destroy everything in its path and does not build nests. They are nomads going from one place to another, finding their food source. Once everything is devoured in their path, they move on to the next place. Their size is small, but it is their numbers that make them deadly. They can swarm an animal, stinging and biting and leaving it dead within minutes.

This is the only ant in the world that could devour a human. Of course, you have to stay still and let the beasts do their work, so the likelihood of dying by this horrible creature is extremely low. Typically, the Siafu ant will perceive you as a threat, sting, and bite you until you are unable to do anything, and then leave you to die rather than leave you as a bone.

It does not mean you should stay in the path of a swarm of Siafu ants or allow them to crawl all over you. These ants want to find food, which is plants, so if you get out of the way, they are going to keep devouring the plants they eat and ignore you.

As long as you keep moving, knock them off, or kill them, you are going to be able to get away alive.

Unfortunately, there are people allergic to ants, including the Siafu, so you are more likely to die from an allergic reaction or infection of the wound site than a swarm.

You can seek medical care and should if you encounter multiple bites.

Siafu Emergency Care

Get out of the swarm's way by getting into a vehicle or running out of their path.

1. Monitor yourself for any allergic reaction to the venom this ant produces.

2. Clean the bite/sting area with soap and water.

3. Apply an anti-itch medication.

4. Take an antihistamine.

5. Cover the wound area.

6. Continue to monitor yourself for a delayed allergic reaction.

7. Keep the wound covered, apply anti-itch cream whenever you feel the itch, continue taking an antihistamine to reduce the pain and itchy feeling.

8. Seek medical care if an allergic reaction presents.

Your best defense against the bite/sting is to ensure you are providing proper care without causing an infection in the wound site. If you develop a fever, pus around the wound, or a spreading of pain, seek medical attention. Any infection needs to be treated by a professional to prevent any chance of death due to infection. You are more likely to develop an infection or gangrene from an improperly treated wound than you are to die from the swarm, mainly because you can keep moving and get away from the beasts.

Fire Ant

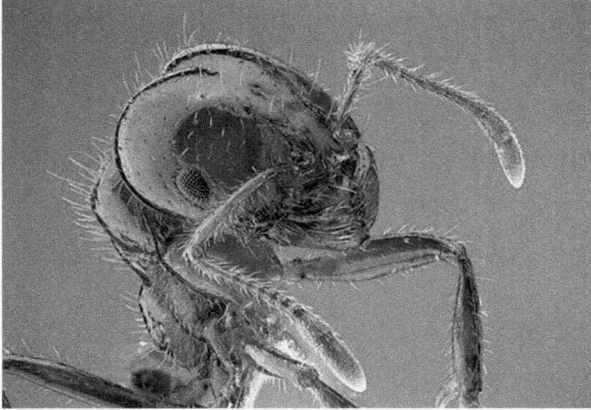

Fire ants are aggressive when provoked. They produce a pheromone that will call other ants in their colony, which means you can go from seeing one ant to multiple ants in moments. A fire ant sting is excruciating and can lead to swelling, puss, and redness of the wound area. People have developed allergic reactions to fire ants and died from anaphylactic shock.

There are over 200 species of fire ants in the world. They belong to the genus Solenopsis and the order Hymenoptera. Common names include red imported, southern, black imported, red harvester, ginger, and tropical fire ants. They are stinging ants. 13 states in the US have a species of the fire ant. They are about a half-inch in length and red to brown in color. They build mounds, so it is easy to spot an area that may be infested with fire ants.

According to Medical News Today, fire ant venom has 46 proteins that typically irritate the skin but does not lead to a significant problem. However, testing has shown enough fire ant venom can affect the nervous system. You will feel a fire ant sting/bite. The pain in most people is short-lived but can produce a pimple-like a wound and an itching sensation. The itching will increase over the next couple of days, as your immune system fights the offending venom. Providing you do not open the wounds; the stings will heal without treatment. However, some will become puss-filled or blistered that could lead to an infection.

The important thing about fire ants is that some people are allergic, and they can have a severe reaction. The sting can swell, burn, itch, and the venom can lead to trouble breathing, swelling of the throat or tongue, dizziness, confusion, and loss of consciousness. Untreated allergic reactions can cause the body to go into shock, and eventually, death can occur.

An allergic reaction is relatively rare. However, if you are allergic to bees and other insects, you should avoid fire ants and seek immediate medical assistance if bitten/stung. You can monitor yourself or others for an allergic reaction to ensure you do not have a severe reaction. There are two levels of care, depending on you or someone else's reaction to fire ant bites.

Emergency Care for Fire Ant Bites

If you are stung, you want to monitor yourself or the stung person for an allergic reaction. Anytime there are multiple stings from multiple assailants, you will want to seek medical attention. The more bites/stings you experience, the more venom from the ant delivers to your system. It can be extremely uncomfortable or lead to more severe health issues.

1. Wash the area of the sting with soap and water.

2. Apply a topical anti-itch cream.

3. If there is swelling around the bite/sting wound, use a cold compress to help limit the swelling.

4. Cover the area to prevent scratching and infection.

5. Repeat these steps until the problem is alleviated.

The pain can be uncomfortable, as well as the itch. You can use an antihistamine to help with the itching and a pain reliever for the pain. However, if the affected person starts to experience any trouble breathing or heart palpitations, you should seek a medical professional.

The second level of care comes in if there is an allergic reaction or too many bites from these ants. A medical professional will examine the blood count for any infection, monitor breathing, and heart rate. If there appears to be no reaction, then a person can be released and monitored for the next 72 hours. However, if complications arise, an antibiotic may be administered, along with medication, to help a patient breathe. If you are not close to medical care at the time an allergic reaction presents, help keep the patient calm, call for help, keep the person immobile, check to make sure no other bites/stings are occurring, and provide CPR if necessary.

Bullet Ant

Some people liken the bullet ant bite to that of a gunshot, hence the common name. This ant lives in South America. It is also called the

24-hour ant because of people's reactions to the bites. Experts say you can feel the pain of the bite for around 24 hours before the wound begins to ooze pus. It is also stated that it would take 2,250 stings before the ants would deliver enough venom to kill a 165-pound human. Those who have been bitten say the pain is excruciating. However, once the toxin leaves the body and all the adrenaline is still in the system, you feel fantastic. Personally, finding out would not be the best option. You never know what allergies you might have, and you definitely do not want to step in a pile of a thousand of these ants to prove how many stings you need to become lethally injected with their neurotoxin.

The emergency care for such an ant is to ride the pain. There is little to do other than use a pain reliever to help lower the pain felt and allow the wound to excrete pus. Of course, you do want to keep the wound area clean, covered, and monitor it for infection. The worst problem with ants is the potential for infection to set in due to an unclean wound.

1. Use warm soap and water to clean the area.

2. Apply an anti-itch cream to help lower the desire to scratch the area.

3. Use a loose wrapping to cover the wound.

4. Take a pain reliever.

5. Wash the wound every 8 hours, even during the height of pain to keep it clean, particularly as the puss begins to ooze.

6. Keep it loosely covered.

7. Monitor the area for any infection.

8. Seek medical attention if you feel the wound is not recovering, if pain persists, or if an allergic reaction presents.

Florida Harvester Ant

As discussed in a previous section, harvester ants can be extremely uncomfortable if they bite or sting. They can also be considered one of the deadliest ants in the world due to their venom; although, it would take a significant amount to kill you or someone else. Children are the most at-risk from these ants because they are smaller, so it takes less venom to harm children.

Florida harvester ants are not limited to one state. They are located in North, South, and Central America. According to Lake Norman Pest control, the venom delivered by harvester ants can be as lethal as a Cobra bite. Luckily, these ants do not bite or sting unless provoked, so if you see many ants carrying food around to their colony, do not try to kill them with your feet. Avoid them and call for pest control to eradicate the colony.

Medical Care when Florida Harvester Ants Are Involved

One ant is not going to be lethal; however, an entire upset colony can be deadly to a human.

1. Get away from the ants.

2. Knock them off your body or the person who is being stung.

3. When clear of the ants, check the health condition of the one stung. Is there any trouble breathing? The heart rate may be

heightened due to the flight or fight response (adrenaline rush) experienced.

4. If no immediate, life-threatening symptoms are noted, clean the sting areas with soap and water.

5. Apply an anti-itch cream.

6. If possible, cover the welts with bandages.

7. Continue to monitor a person for any life-threatening symptoms or infection of the wound areas.

Seek immediate medical professionals if an allergic reaction presents, if hundreds of bites/stings occurred, or if the individual is a child, elder, or at-risk person.

Once the medical care is provided, get pest control out to the area to prevent further issues.

Bullhorn Acacia Ant

The bullhorn acacia ant is similar to a wasp in structure. While smaller, it packs a wasp-like punch if stung. The ant will inject venom that brings on a burning sensation. In some people, this ant has caused anaphylactic shock. Interestingly, it has been found that in small doses, this venom can aid depression and asthma. Some research combines venom with other known chemicals to help treat both conditions.

Your best move is to avoid this ant when you see it. Do not threaten it or remain nearby to be stung. If you are stung, provide the following medical treatment.

1. Get away from the area, and look out for any other colonies of these ants. Stay away from them to avoid being stung again.

2. Wash the stung area with soap and warm water.

3. Apply an anti-itch cream.

4. Cover the welt.

5. Monitor the welt for any rash, increased pain or swelling.

6. If a person begins to show signs of breathing difficulties or an erratic heartbeat, call 911 or get them to the nearest medical facility.

7. Provide CPR if the person stops breathing or the heart stops.

8. If no allergic reaction presents, continue to clean and monitor the stung area until it heals.

One of the most significant issues is the infection of the wound area if it becomes an open sore or is not kept clean.

Green Tree Ant

The green tree ant lives in Australia and parts of Southeast Asia. It is also called a weaver ant because it will nest on trees and leaves. They stitch their nests together to form a colony home. One colony can have at least a half-million ants in it. Green ants do not sting; they bite. Their bites are painful and, while not said to contain venom, can lead to infection. Green tree ants are also harvested for their medical advantages, including in the treatment of stomach aches and fertility.

One bite from this ant is not going to kill you; even a few dozen will not. However, like with most insects, if you sustain hundreds or thousands of bites, they could become lethal. The most concerning aspect of any bite will be an infection or allergic reaction. At most, people experience pain for several days, coupled with itching and a little localized swelling around the bite areas.

Medical Treatment

Unless you or another person experiences an allergic reaction to the ants' bites, you will not have to call 911 or get to a nearby medical facility.

1. Get away from the ant colony.

2. Get all the ants off you or the other person as quickly as possible.

3. Clean the bites.

4. Apply an anti-itch cream.

5. Cover the bites.

6. Take an antihistamine for the itch and a pain reliever for any pain.

7. Monitor yourself up to 8 hours for any allergic reaction.

8. Repeat the cleaning, itch cream, and medication as needed until the wound(s) heal.

An infection can occur, so you need to keep the bite areas clean and monitor for any puss excretions, redness, swelling, or other reactions.

If you suspect there is an infection, seek your doctor. Most infections, when caught early, take treatment of antibiotics and will alleviate any issues. Prolonged infections where gangrene sets in can be life-threatening.

Jack Jumper Ant

The last ant to discuss is the Jack jumper ant, which is similar to a sting like a small scorpion. Research states there have been at least 4 deaths by a Jack jumper ant since 1980. It is not the sting that can kill a person. Instead, it is the shock, heart attack, inflammation, and irritation that can present due to a sting. The sting from a Jack jumper weakens the immune system, and in some people has been known to cause irregular heartbeats and even death. A person who is young, elderly, or prone to illness is most susceptible to Jack jumper's effects.

Most cases end with a painful bite, lasting discomfort for a few days, and the need to monitor for infection. However, you should see a doctor if bitten by one of these ants.

The jack jumper ant lives in Australia. They can be 10 to 15 millimeters in length and they have a black body with orange or brown pincers and limbs. The Jack jumper will grab their prey by the pincers and then bend to sting them. They are aggressive and have a hopping motion. They live in vegetation like gardens.

Symptoms
- Localized swelling usually results from a sting.

- Pain around the sting area is also common.

- The swelling and pain can last for several days.

Allergic Reactions

- Difficulty breathing

- Swelling of the tongue and throat

- A persistent cough

- Vomiting

- Abdominal pain

- Loss of consciousness

- Swelling in the face, eyes, and lips

- Hives or welts

Anaphylaxis is actually common among those in Australia and other areas where this ant can be found. A survey showed 2 to 3 percent of people have localized allergic reactions, and about half of those who show a reaction have life-threatening symptoms. An Australian website states there have been several recorded deaths by Jack jumper ants, even in recent years. The allergy does not appear immediately. In about 70% of people with an allergy to the ant venom, the reaction will make it look as if they have been stung multiple times.

It is best to have a management protocol in place if one is known to have an allergic reaction to these ants (usually only a known allergy occurs after the first sting). Royal Adelaide Hospital, Monash Hospital, Melbourne, and Royal Hobart Hospitals all have treatment therapies that have shown a 90% effective rate in patients.

Avoid the ants. Have pest control in the area. Never work in a garden without gloves and boots. These ants are known to have tough pincers that can go through clothing.

Medical Treatment for Jack Jumper Ant Stings

Due to the higher than normal allergic reaction to Jack jumper ant stings, it is best to be prepared for the potential situation.

1. If this ant bites you, quickly get away from any potential nest area and try to kill the ant.

2. If you have any known allergies, such as to bee stings, have an adrenaline autoinjector like the Epi-Pen on hand. Adrenaline should be considered the most effective treatment if you have any on hand.

3. Whether you have an adrenaline shot or not, immediately head to the nearest medical facility. Do not wait to see if an allergic reaction will take place. It is better to be on your way than to wait and not make it; especially, since some hospitals can be quite far from a person's location in Australia.

4. Keep track of the number of stings sustained, more stings than one can lead to a reaction within a few hours.

5. During the drive, if someone can help, get the sting area clean.

6. At the hospital or medical facility, the professionals will clean the area, ask about your symptoms, and provide proper treatment, which may include an adrenaline shot, then an antibiotic to help with any potential infection. They may also provide a pain reliever that will not interfere with your heart rate.

If you do not show signs of anaphylaxis, you may be released and told to monitor your condition from home or your accommodation. If any further reactions occur, such as hives, extreme pain, or heart troubles, you will need to return to the medical facility, or you will be kept for observation if these issues arise while you are at the care center.

It is suggested that you:

- Carry a mobile or satellite phone with you if you are going to be in the outback or rainforest in Australia, New Zealand, or Southeast Asia.

- Do not travel alone in remote areas.

- When going into places that Jack jumper ants are common, take an antihistamine before going out. An antihistamine will relieve mild symptoms but will not prevent a severe allergic reaction.

If you have a known allergy, your physician may prescribe an adrenaline injector plus blood pressure or heart medication to treat a severe allergic reaction. There is no skin test for this ant; therefore, unless you are stung, you may not know you have an allergy to this ant.

SECTION 3

Animal Bites

Animal bites are rare, but not unheard of, which is why you should know what to do in an emergency. In fact, some "dangerous animal" lists do not contain all animals. Instead, they are a combination of reptiles, fish, and mammals. So, this section will look at the most dangerous animals that fit these categories, why they might attack, and the emergency care you need to implement when something happens. Your immediate first aid can be the difference between life and death for someone.

Chapter 8

Stampeding, Biting, Stinging and More

In this chapter, we will look at the list of the top eight animals, fish, and reptiles to avoid. The key to being safe around these creatures is to know where they live and when you might encounter them, plus what to do in an emergency situation.

Cape Buffalo

The Cape buffalo is a nearly six-foot animal that weighs almost 2,000 pounds. It lives in sub-Saharan Africa. For anyone living in this area or wishing to visit, you definitely want to be careful. They are not going to bite, but their horns can gorge, and their heavyweight can trample a person. Cape buffalo are usually mild creatures, but when threatened or wounded, they can become

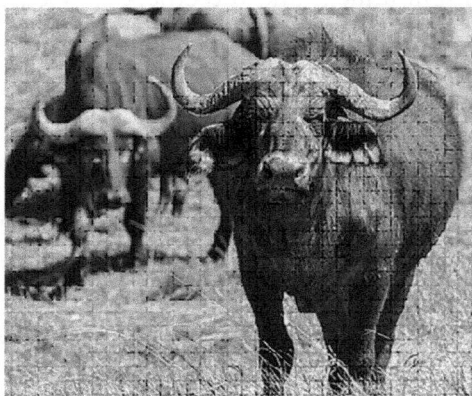

the "black death" that will kill you or someone in your party. They are known for killing hunters. They are also not hesitant in charging a vehicle.

1. Do not engage in threatening behavior when around a Cape buffalo or their herd.

2. If something causes a stampede or attack, attempt to get inside a vehicle or high off the ground.

3. If an injury occurs, provide medical care based on the issue.

Two things are likely with Cape buffalo: trampling or gorging from their massive horns. A person can also be thrown as the buffalo uses the horns to stab and then toss the victim.

Handling a Trampling

1. Do not attempt to distract the buffalo. The herd or individual will move on when the perceived threat is gone. Wait for the area to become empty.

2. Immediately check to make sure the person is breathing, and the heart is still beating.

3. Assess the injuries if they are breathing, and the heart is beating. Is the person conscious? Are there any immediate signs of head injury or broken bones? If the person can speak, ask questions to determine any possible injury.

4. Immobilize any broken bone with a splint. If there is a fear of spinal damage, use a stretcher. Make sure one person holds

the head and neck still while two people roll the person onto the stretcher (if you have enough people to help).

5. If the person is not conscious, do a physical examination for bruising, cuts, gorges, or broken bones. Treat the person as if they have a spinal injury.

6. If a person is not breathing or has no heartbeat, provide CPR methods, while getting the person into a vehicle and transported to the nearest medical facility as soon as possible.

A head injury can be fatal, and you may not be able to resuscitate a person. Additionally, if one of the horns has pierced or severed a major artery, there may be nothing you can do.

If the horns or broken bones have caused a severe bleeding issue, you will need to address the loss of blood before any other concerns.

7. Applying a tourniquet may cause the loss of a limb, but it is better than the loss of life. You need to ensure the tourniquet is tight enough to stop the blood flow or minimize it. Do not attempt to sew the area.

8. Once you have the tourniquet in place, you still need to pack the wound with gauze to soak up any blood.

9. Wrap the wound once it is packed with gauze. Keep the wound wrapped to prevent any dirt or particles from getting into the area and causing an infection. The wound is already a mess from the attack, but at this point, you need to

administer quick care that will ensure quick transportation to a qualified professional. Do not worry about cleaning the wound; just get the blood loss stopped.

10. Treat other injuries that could lead to life-threatening conditions. Minor issues can wait; it is better to seek medical attention as quickly as possible.

11. Once you have the person in a condition to transport them, seek medical care quickly.

Due to the remote locations, many of these injuries occur, it is unlikely that an emergency medical team would get to you fast enough. It is better to attempt transportation to the nearest emergency location.

Cone Snail

A cone snail is a tropical gastropod that lives in Hawaii, Indonesia, and the Caribbean. They have a brown and white marbled shell that can be seen when scuba diving or snorkeling. They like to be near coral reefs, rocks, or along sandy shoals. The cone snail has teeth. You want to avoid picking up this animal or, worse, stepping on it. These harpoon-style teeth have a conotoxin (venom) that is poisonous to humans at a high dose. The toxin like that of scorpion venom attacks the central nervous system, and there is no antivenom.

If you do sustain a bite:

1. Immediately get out of the water.

2. Alert anyone nearby to the injury.

3. Immobilize the limb that sustained the bite to prevent the spread of the toxin in your body.

4. Monitor yourself for a toxic reaction while you obtain transportation to the nearest medical facility. If no one is around to help, you will need to get yourself to the emergency care location, as quickly as possible, and with as little panic and movement as possible.

5. Do not wait to get to a medical professional. Do not move around or massage the area, as this will cause the toxin to spread.

6. Depending on your symptoms, you may be released after a professional treat the wound and any pain. If your symptoms are more severe, you may be admitted and given an IV of fluids to keep you hydrated.

7. If you are released, keep the area clean, monitor the wound for any sign of infection, and follow your doctor's orders.

Symptoms can include:

- Local pain

- Local welt

- Nausea

- Vomiting

- Severe pain radiating throughout the body

- Paralysis

- Convulsions

- Heart irregularities

- Breathing troubles, including respiratory distress

Not all bites will deliver enough venom to kill a human; however, you do not want to wait and allow the venom to spread throughout your body.

Golden Poison Dart Frog

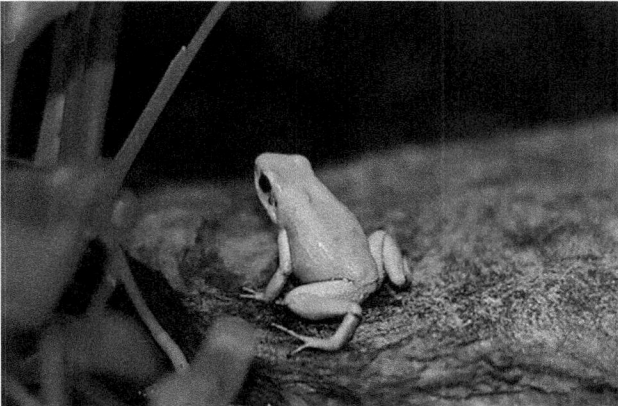

This dart frog is named for its golden skin color. There are several poison dart frogs, which live in northern South America, typically, in the Amazon rainforest and along Colombia's Pacific Coast. It is a two-inch long amphibian. The point is—this amphibian has a batrachotoxin. Just two micrograms of the toxin can kill one adult human. All you have to do is touch this frog to become poisoned. The poison glands are in the skin, so brushing up against it or touching it can disperse the toxin.

Do not touch it. If for some reason, you brush up against it or it hops on your bare skin, you will need to seek emergency care.

Emergency Treatment for Golden Poison Dart Frog

Due to the lethality of these frogs, you do not want to delay in getting medical attention.

1. Have a mobile or satellite phone with you when you go into areas where these frogs are common.

2. Take an antihistamine before going out into the jungle. It will not stop a poison reaction; however, it can help keep the airway clear, even marginally so, should an issue arise.

3. If you have a known allergy, carry an adrenaline autoinjector with you. While the poison does not lead to an allergic reaction such as a bee sting, adrenaline can help restart the heart due to shock or paralysis from the toxin.

4. Never go alone into an area with these frogs.

5. Call for immediate help if you encounter a poison dart frog.

6. Make sure you or the person affected is no longer near the frog or others for the second round of poison.

7. Keep the person immobile and calm, to help prevent the spread of the poison and to prevent shock-related reactions.

8. Administer oxygen, if you have any with you, should breathing distress present itself.

9. If the patient's heart stops beating or they are no longer capable of breathing on their own, start administering the proper CPR techniques. For paralysis of the diaphragm, you will need to tilt the head back and lift the chin to open the airway and provide steady breaths.

10. If the heart stops, use an AED or use hand compressions to attempt to get the heart started again.

11. Continue to provide CPR until medical help arrives.

12. If you do not have to provide CPR, keep the patient calm, try to minimize any shock, and using a stretcher or other immobility device, get the patient to the nearest help. You can also wait for help if it arrives faster than you can get out of the area.

Never wait to see if a person sustained enough of poisoning to be life-threatening. React as if the person has had a lethal dose and get to a care facility as quickly as possible.

Jellyfish – Box, Man-o-War, Lion's Mane, Sea Wasp, Irukandji

Jellyfish are simplistic creatures, with only a few cells that make up their ability to live and survive in the ocean. One of the adaptations they have is to sting their prey. Most jellyfish are found in groups, floating on the ocean currents, so if one looks from a vantage point into the sea, it is easy to spot them and stay out of their path. Sometimes, they wash up on shore but do not mistake their death on land to mean they are no longer lethal or painful. Stepping on, their stingers can be dangerous.

Some jellyfish are more dangerous than others. Of course, multiple stings, like with ants, can lead to death; however, others are lethal with just one stinging you. The Box jellyfish is considered the most dangerous, and there are multiple species of this jellyfish. The box jellyfish tend to live in Indo-Pacific waters near Australia, Japan, and Southeast Asia. Their structure is box-like with 15 tentacles. The body plus tentacles can grow up to 15 feet, so you may not see the body, but you can feel the sting. All tentacles have nematocysts (stinging cells) that contain toxins. The Portuguese man-o-war, lion's mane, sea wasp, and Irukandji are the other lethal jellyfish you do not want to encounter while in the water.

The Irukandji is a few small jellyfish, possible to see by the naked eye, yet you might not see it until you have been stung multiple times.

Symptoms from one of these jellyfish stings:

- Heart attack

- Central nervous system shut down

- Pain at the site

If stung, a victim can go into shock, have a heart attack, and possibly drown before reaching a boat or shore. Survivors have been able to get to the hospital quick enough to get an antidote for box jellyfish stings, but pain can last for weeks, and scars, from the tentacles, can remain for life.

The Irukandji is said to have a toxin that is 100 times that of a cobra, and multiple stings are deadly. Symptoms include:

- Muscle cramps

- Kidney pain

- Burning sensations

- Headache

- Vomiting

- Irregular heartbeat

Sea wasp deaths number in the 5,500s. The tentacles, like most box jellyfish, are over 10 feet in length, with many darts or stingers. One dart is said to have enough toxin to kill 60 people, theoretically.

The man-o-war can have long tentacles, and a purple and pink, with a blue tint body, remains close to the surface. It travels in a large group, and that is why it can be deadly. Too many stings from this jellyfish relative can release too much toxin in the body. Just one cannot kill you, but since they travel in packs, they can be very dangerous.

The Lion's mane jellyfish can reach 8 feet in body size and over 100 feet in tentacle length. While one may not be deadly, multiple stings can undoubtedly lead to death. You do not want to get trapped in one of these because, at the very least, the sting will be quite painful for days.

Treatment of Jellyfish Stings

Depending on the offending jellyfish, you may need to seek immediate medical attention. We will discuss both non-lethal and potentially deadly stings and what care to provide.

1. First, if you notice any jellyfish washed up on shore or floating near your boat, do not get in the water.

2. Always keep one person on the boat as a lookout for potential dangers and to help in a medical emergency.

3. If stung, alert the person onboard or onshore to the issue. They should immediately call for emergency assistance if you are in an area with box jellyfish or other deadly species. It is better to call for assistance and not need it than to call too late to get help.

4. Swim away from the jellyfish and try to avoid any others in the area. Do not remain still and hope the jellyfish will move on; it is powered mostly by the current, so you must swim away.

5. Attempt to get to shore or on the boat. If it was a highly dangerous jellyfish-like, the box jelly, the person onshore or onboard, may need to come to get you or someone else. Never swim to rescue someone else. Use the boat to maneuver closer or take a water vehicle from shore. If you are in the

water, do not try to get close to the affected person, but swim away and monitor the water to avoid getting stung.

6. Apply vinegar to the sting, unless other more troubling health troubles are apparent. Vinegar will help relieve the sting. According to many sources, peeing will not help. However, they suggest that peeing will release more toxins from the jellyfish if it is still around you. Instead, the idea of peeing on the sting is when you are clear from the stings and potential further stings. Still, it is better to use vinegar or a similar product to alleviate the burn and pain from the stings.

7. If a sea wasp, Irukandji, or species of box jellyfish is the culprit of the stinging, you may need to use CPR. Check to see if the person is breathing and if the heart is pumping. If a heart attack occurred, provide CPR.

8. Make sure help is on the way, or someone else is helping you get the injured person to the nearest help.

While a sting may not be lethal, you do not want to change the toxin from spreading and turning lethal. Box jellyfish are the most lethal, but an allergic reaction or compromised immune system can lead to death. Older, younger, or at-risk people can die from the above jellyfish stings. Treat any sting as potentially lethal if you are in the Indo-Pacific region, near Japan, or Southeast Asia.

Black Mamba

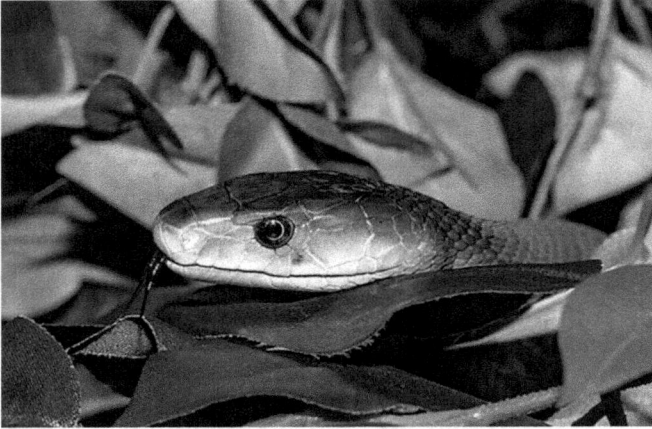

The black mamba is a snake and considered extremely dangerous. Rattlesnake, boomslang, and king cobra bites are dangerous, due to their poison and can lead to death, but the black mamba is quicker and more likely to strike. The black mamba is found in rocky areas of Africa. The fastest snake alive, it grows up to 14 feet in length and can move 12.5 miles per hour. As with most snakes, it attacks when threatened. They also bite repeatedly when threatened, which is why they can be lethal. One bite has enough neuro and cardiotoxin combination to kill ten people. Antivenom is needed within 20 minutes of a bite. Studies indicate bites when they occur, are nearly 100 percent lethal. There is less than a 0.01 percent chance of a bite not being lethal within 20 minutes.

Before going anywhere this snake lives, you will need to recognize what it looks like. Despite its name as the "black" mamba, it does not have to be black in appearance. It can be a gray color. It likes rocks and trees.

Emergency Protocol for Black Mamba Bites

The best thing to do is stay away from its habitat. Do not go climbing or walking in a place you might encounter this snake. If you are, make sure you have a few things on hand.

1. Never go alone.

2. Carry a mobile or satellite phone to ensure you can call for help.

3. Wear high calf boots to avoid being bitten.

4. Do not place your hands near crevices, rocks, or trees.

5. Observe the area before moving around.

6. If a snake bites someone in your party, try to render it unable to bite again. A second bite would most certainly be lethal to an adult human.

7. Remember that most snakes, even when shot or injured, do not immediately die; you are better off severing the head.

8. The affected person will need antivenom within 20 minutes.

9. The poison will spread throughout the body, affecting the heart, causing paralysis, and making it impossible to breathe the longer it is in the body.

10. A tourniquet will not stop the spread of the poison, although pop culture would have you believe it is appropriate to use one. You should also not try to suck the venom out or in any

way touch the bite area. You could cause an infection that would bring on the long term effects.

11. Rather than a tourniquet, make sure the area is safe and get the person immobile. The worst part about a snake bite is the fear of death, which can lead to hysteria and movement. A pounding heart will bring the toxin through the body quicker than someone resting.

12. It is not true that a prone position will keep the poison from circulating. Instead, a prone and immobile position is to provide CPR quicker if it becomes necessary. You want the heart to do as little work as possible to help keep the person alive.

13. Do not pause in getting help or administering CPR when it is necessary.

14. You have a 20-minute window to meet up with medical professionals and get the antivenom.

It is unlikely a person will survive a bite if antivenom is not administered within the 20-minute window. Unfortunately, the antivenom is not something you can buy to carry in your first aid kit. The cost of production is too high for it to be affordable or sold on the private market.

While the black mamba is undoubtedly the most dangerous snake in Africa, it is by no means the only deadly snake. Rattlesnakes, saw-scaled viper, habu, yellow chin snake, boomslang, Australian cobra, banded krait, king cobra, and taipan are all deadly snakes to humans.

In fact, the inland or western Taipan has a mix of toxins, including neurotoxins, procoagulants, myotoxins, and taipoxins that will cause paralysis within moments, respiratory issues, hemorrhaging of the blood vessels and muscle damage—if you survive.

Not all snakes have an antivenom or one that is widespread enough to get to in an emergency. Depending on the type of snake, death can occur in ten minutes to an hour, depending on the medical aid provided. The best thing to do is to follow the steps above to make the person immobile and to reduce the possibility of the poison spreading too fast through their system that antivenom or hospital treatment would be too late.

Never ignore a snake bite, primarily, in areas with known deadly snakes. It could be the difference between life and death if you hesitate to call for help or do not consider the bite dangerous. Reactions can take a little time to show, depending on the type of snake, but once the poison spreads, it is hard to ensure life will prevail over the toxin. Additionally, snakes like the Taipan, which have more than one toxin in their poison, are deadlier than those with just one toxin.

Saltwater Crocodile

Crocodiles are reptiles, yet they still wind up on many animal lists because their bites can be extremely deadly. Unlike the snake, a crocodile does not have poison—just sharp teeth—to tear a person apart. Death commonly occurs due to blood loss as a result of a crocodile attack.

While the saltwater crocodile is mentioned here, you should not forget the alligators in Florida are just as deadly as crocodiles. The reason crocodiles are on the list and alligators are just mentioned is due to the aggressiveness of the species. Crocodiles are incredibly aggressive, easily angered, and short-tempered. The saltwater crocodile is the largest of all crocodiles, and even more massive than most alligators. They live in the Indo-Pacific regions, including Australia, India, and Vietnam. They grow up to 23 feet in length and can weigh more than 2,000 pounds. The crocodiles in these regions are responsible for hundreds of deaths each year, far more deaths than attributes to sharks per year.

Saltwater crocodiles are agile swimmers, and just because they prefer saltwater doesn't mean they cannot survive in freshwater. A bite by this crocodile provides 3,700 pounds per square inch of pressure.

Preventing a crocodile attack:

You can avoid being crocodile food.

- Stay out of the waters in the Indo-Pacific region.

- Keep an eye out if you are near any water.

- Do not have any wounds and do not stand in the water when fishing.

Emergency Care for a Crocodile Bite
Blood loss is the biggest reason for death by a crocodile.

1. A crocodile, when angered, will attack. Depending on what is closest to the mouth, a bite can cause severe a limb, rip through the abdomen, or, worse, cause instant death by decapitation.

2. If a bite occurs, anyone in the area must immediately call for emergency personnel.

3. Attempt to get away from the crocodile or help the person being attacked getaway (if you can do so safely). Poking the crocodile in the eyes can provide temporary relief from a bite and hopefully get the person to safety. It is also said that the more you fight back and try to harm the crocodile, the more likely they are to release you, realizing they do not want to keep the fight going. Smacking the sensitive snout can also help.

4. Whatever you do, do not put yourself in a position that will gain a bite. It is hard to watch someone else get attacked, but you can only help if you remain unharmed.

5. Crocodiles can take their prey with them and may not leave the area. Do not get in the water or attempt to retrieve an injured person until you are 100 percent certain there are no crocodiles in the area.

6. Do what you can to remain out of harm's way and rescue the person from the water or land.

7. Once safety has been reached, it is time to assess the injuries and find the worst one and start triage.

8. Typically, blood loss is the primary concern because too much blood loss leads to shock, organ shut down, and eventually death.

9. Use a tourniquet on any limb that is bleeding excessively. If an artery is punctured, the flow will be extreme, and only the best tourniquet will stop the excessive loss. Pack the wounds with gauze to help steep the flow and then tightly wind bandage material around the packed wound.

10. Never release a tourniquet or remove gauze already packed into a wound. Attempt to tighten a tourniquet more if extreme blood loss continues. Add packed gauze over the wound. Try to apply pressure or have someone help to keep the pressure on the worst wound.

11. There may be several wounds, which may require a few tourniquets. Remember, you need to stop all extreme blood loss to prevent death.

12. Leave the minimal wounds or shallow bites in favor of keeping pressure on the areas of high blood loss or administering CPR. Chest compressions may not be effective if pressing on the heart causes more blood to leave through the wounds.

13. Continue CPR and minimizing blood loss until emergency personnel arrives to take over.

The longer it takes to stop the blood and get professionals on the scene, the higher the danger of death will be from a crocodile attack.

Lastly, attempting to shoot a crocodile during an attack can lead to the death of the person in danger. A crocodile has very thick skin, so while you do want to make it think a person is not worth the fight, be careful in your attempts at helping someone or you from further damage.

Tsetse Fly Parasites

The tsetse fly is something we could have discussed in the flying insect chapter on bees and wasps. However, it is not the fly that causes deadly harm to a human. It is the parasite they carry. A tsetse fly bite can deliver a protozoan (single-celled) parasite into your skin. Trypanosomes (the parasites) call sleeping sickness and meningitis. Left untreated, these parasites can kill.

Unfortunately, tsetse flies are only 0.7 inches in size, so they are not very large, and you may be bitten without realizing it. These flies live in the Congo, Sudan, and Angola. You should avoid being out at night. You also want to wear neutral colors because blue and other bright colors can attract flies. Do not go into bushes or wear permethrin-treated gear.

There is no medication or vaccine for these parasites. It is in treating the symptoms at a hospital that may help a person survive a parasitic infection.

Medical professionals will prescribe a course of treatment based on the infection and stage of the disease. You will need to seek medical attention if you suspect you are experiencing any parasitic infection, particularly from the parasite living in tsetse flies. Suramin, melarsoprol, nifurtimox, and eflornithine may be prescribed during the treatment of these parasites. The CDC is the only place that will have treatment protocols, and most are not available in the US. The reason the treatment is not available is that the US does not have these flies. It is rare to see a parasitic infection in the US. However, it is not impossible since someone can visit a place with the flies and come back with an infection without knowing it.

Emergency Care

Due to the delay in symptoms, a person can be infected without realizing it. The symptoms include:

- Headache

- Nausea

- Personality change

- Weight loss

- Irritability

- Seizures

- Slurred speech

- Difficulty walking

- Sleeping more or developing insomnia

Death can occur within a few weeks or months, depending on the symptoms of the African sleeping sickness one shows.

If you experience any of these symptoms and have visited an area the tsetse fly is known to inhabit, do not hesitate to speak with a doctor and have a test to see if you are infected.

There is little you can do at home, unless a seizure or difficulty walking causes a secondary issue, like heart attack, hitting your head, or something else.

Treat any issue that arises with an appropriate medical response and then get yourself tested for any underlying cause like the parasite.

Sharks

Sharks are definitely a fish, but they fall into a dangerous and deadly category, albeit not as dangerous as other "animals" mentioned in this category. There are, on average, 16 shark attacks per year in the United States. According to the worldwide shark attack data from the Florida Museum at the University of Florida. On average, about 140 shark attacks happen worldwide, where 64 are unprovoked, 41 are provoked, and 12 are boat attacks.

An unprovoked attack is often a case of mistaken identity by the shark who is hunting in the dawn or dusk hours, attempting to get a full sea lion or seal meal and encounters a surfer instead. Provoked attacks are those where someone intentionally irritates a shark. About a decade or more ago, a boy pulled on a nurse shark's tail. The shark whipped around and took the boy's arm in its mouth. Nurse sharks are docile creatures but they do have serrated teeth. The shark locked onto the boy and would not let go. The shark died because the boy just couldn't leave the poor, docile shark alone. They are actually one of only a few sharks that can rest on the bottom of the ocean floor. Most sharks need to swim to breathe continuously.

Sharks are by nature predators. They will attack when threatened, hungry, or due to aggressive behaviors. Individual sharks are more dangerous than others. Great white, tiger and bull sharks are the top three most dangerous sharks in the world. A whale shark, which is a shark, is enormous, but only dangerous if you get knocked around by its size.

There are other sharks, like reef and lemon sharks that can be harmful too, in the right conditions, but their attacks are rarer than the top three.

You can prevent a shark attack by staying out of the water during the times they tend to feed because they come close to shore during those hours. Stay out of grassy areas and watch for sharks around reefs when snorkeling or scuba diving.

The US has a bull, tiger, and great white sharks. Tiger sharks hunt mostly on the Pacific side around Hawaii. At the same time, the other two can be found on the Atlantic and Pacific coasts. Australia and South Africa are also highly common areas to see all three. However, tiger and great white sharks are more common.

Interestingly enough, bull sharks have been found to swim up freshwater rivers.

What to do During a Shark Attack

If you are a bystander onshore, the very first thing you need to do is make sure everyone is alerted to the attack. Get everyone out of the water. If lifeguards are on duty at the beach, they will have the equipment to make this happen and be on hand for the emergency. However, not all beaches have lifeguards, so you may be the one who spots the situation first and needs to get everyone out of the water.

Someone, if anyone else is around, will need to take charge. Typically, those with first aid and CPR training will take command. If that is you, then get everyone out of the water, and delegate someone to call for emergency personnel. Either you or someone else will need to get first aid kits and any other emergency equipment to the beach.

A coordinated rescue is necessary to get the person out of the water unless the shark has let go, and the person can swim to a boat or to shore.

Sharks will typically bite once and determine they have not gotten a fleshy seal or sea lion or other prey.

However, blood loss can cause shock, and the person may drown if not rescued from the water. The blood in the water can attract more sharks so stay on a boat or other vessel to ensure you do not get attacked.

Once the person is on the boat or back to shore, it is time to provide emergency care.

1. If the person is conscious, have someone keep the person calm.

2. Address the largest area of blood loss first, while you wait for trained professionals to arrive.

3. You may need to apply a tourniquet, it can be a belt or anything that will tie, and you can tighten down to stop blood loss

4. Keep an eye out for shock as you may need to provide CPR to get the person's heart beating and breathing again.

5. Your first step is to stop the loss of blood to avoid death.

6. Others can also help administer CPR if it is needed.

Your main aim is to keep the person alive until a hospital can be reached or until trained emergency staff arrive on the scene. You never want to endanger yourself or others in attempting to rescue an injured person.

Chapter 9

Animal Attacks
(Bear, Dog, Cat, etc.)

In the United States, being attacked by a bear is something to be concerned about. Bears live in more states than we think. North Carolina, Tennessee, Maine, Alaska, Wyoming, Montana, and Colorado have bears. Most states have black bears, thought to be cute, little creatures, which are not prone to attacking humans. But, as some people have found out, you can be sleeping, non-threatening, and find a black bear biting your head. Yes, the most dangerous bears are still the grizzlies, a type of brown bear. In fact, there are Kodiak brown bears, brown bears, and grizzlies. These bears have enough distinct traits to list them separately in the scientific community. We are going to discuss black and brown bear (including grizzly) attacks separately because brown bears on a whole are more aggressive than black bears. Their size is also more substantial than most black or cinnamon black bears.

Black Bears

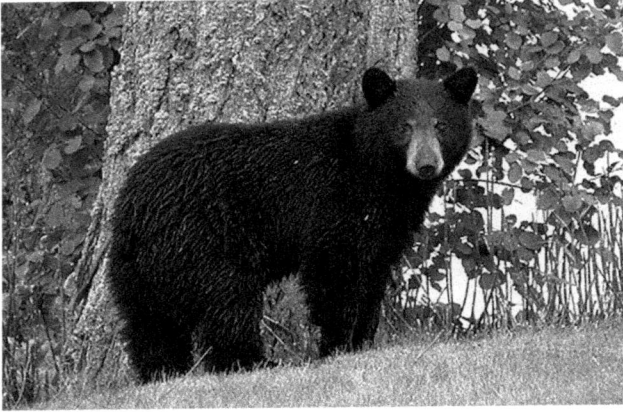

For those who do not live in bear country, it is hard to understand that black bears are not always dark black in color. Many can be cinnamon, with black tones. They usually reach 300 to 400 pounds. They are not known to be aggressive unless threatened, and sometimes they will not react even then. It all depends on their level of fear.

Two people survived an encounter with a black bear unscathed, even the dog was fine. The bear got into the house, wandered around trying to find an exit, and was too scared to even eat a plate of cookies right by the door where it entered the house. Yet, two years later, a college-aged person, camping with friends, their food appropriately stored in the tree, was grabbed by the head in his sleeping bag and had the scars to show what a traumatic experience it was.

You should never approach a bear. If you see a bear, you need to walk away, keep the animal in sight, and move slowly. Like people, bears can perceive eye contact as a threat, so keep it insight, but don't lock eyes. Furthermore, make as much noise as possible and try to look at big as you can. Studies have confirmed that noise and size can help deter a bear.

Do not attempt to shoot a bear. The worst thing you can do is try to kill it, injure it, and ensure a bear attack. They are not easy to kill.

A bear standing on its hindlegs is showing its size. A growl is a sign of aggression. A bear on four paws, with eyes on you, but no growl will probably walk away as long as you remain unthreatening.

What To Do If a Bear Attacks

1. If a bear attacks, it will swipe with its long nails and try to bite. You need to curl into a ball to protect your head and vital organs as best you can. The most damage comes from a bear sinking its teeth or claws into an area that is vital to your survival.

2. Panic and shock can be a factor; however, if you can keep your wits about you, it is better to wait for a break in the attack and attempt to get away. Yes, the concept of playing dead exists because specialists believe if you relax and act dead, the bear will leave you alone. This is not always the case; however, if you are being attacked, it is the better choice. You can also try to make noise, upset the animal, and show it that you are willing to fight back. This method has worked in some instances, and the bear decided the human was not worth the trouble.

3. Do not attempt to run or climb a tree. Black bears can climb. They are also quite fast.

The emergency medical care required after a bear attack will depend on where the animal has injured you or another person. Assessment of the injuries is imperative, but you also want to make sure the bear has indeed left the area before attempting to administer first aid.

Emergency Care

Start by surveying the area. If the bear is gone or distracted, it will be easier for you to get to safety. Most bear attacks happen in the wilderness, which may or may not have cell phone service. If you are in an area with phone coverage, call 911 immediately. The dispatcher will alert the correct people to get medical attention to you. In some instances, you may need to help the injured party out of the wooded area to get medical care quickly. Other times, you may be able to stay where you are and get an airlift from a rescue team.

1. Triage- this is the first step medical professionals use to assess a person's condition. It is meant to do as much as possible to stabilize a person and ready them for more thorough medical treatment.

2. Check for any excessive blood loss. Any limb, abdomen, or another bite that is causing sufficient blood loss can lead to death. The faster the blood is pumping, the quicker a person can expire.

3. Using gauze and bandaging get the blood flow to stop. You may need a tourniquet for severe bites that have injured an

artery or vein. The head is tough and can have copious amounts of blood spilling from even a superficial wound. If the patient is responsive, without confusion, a head wound may not be as bad as it appears. However, you still need to monitor their condition. Blood loss can still affect a person, and damage may be done that you cannot readily see.

4. Once the blood flow is reduced, it will be time to determine other possible injuries. Blood loss can happen due to a broken bone, so you may need to immobilize the broken bone before moving away from the area.

5. Depending on where a wound is, such as near the back, you may need a stretcher to get the person back to a vehicle and to medical care. Even if a person believes they are fine, if you see any sign of injury near the spine, do not let the person walk. If you are only one person, with an injured party, carrying the other person may be your only option. You must do as much as possible to minimize further injury.

Sometimes a person is not responsive. The shock could have rendered them unconscious, a strong knock to the head may have put them to sleep, or the injuries may be severe enough combined with a shock that resuscitation is necessary.

The above steps describe what to do if the person is responsive or if there is significant blood loss. The following will talk you through what to do if blood loss, and breathing and heart stoppage occur.

1. You need to stop blood loss. No one can be resuscitated if they lose too much blood. So, your first priority is to determine how much blood is leaving the body and how you can stop it. A minor injury should be ignored. A gushing artery, use a tourniquet.

2. If blood loss is not an issue, your priority becomes resuming the heart and oxygen to the brain. CPR will be required. If you have an oxygen mask and defibrillator, now is the time to use both. If you do not, then follow the first aid/CPR procedures you learned in your course.

   For those who have not had a CPR course in years, the methods have changed.

3. Tilt the head to open the airway. Check to see if this helps resume breathing; if not, you will need to provide oxygen.

4. Push hard, and push fast on the chest if there is no pulse. You need to deliver 100 compressions per minute.

5. Give two breaths.

6. Resume the hard and fast compressions for another minute.

Ideally, you will hear rib bones break if you are doing CPR correctly. The rib cage is designed to protect the heart, so you must push hard and quickly.

If a pulse is found, you can stop compressions. If breathing resumes, you can stop providing oxygen.

Should the person revive, it will be time to provide first aid for transportation to the nearest medical center. Since you started by calling 911, it is best to assess the person's condition and what you need to do to help them survive until the professionals are reached or arrive.

The damage from a black bear is more likely going to be slashed from very sharp claws and bites. Some people have required extensive stitches and skin grafts, while a few have suffered lost fingers or limbs. Jaws can be broken, and skulls can be crushed, but still, people survive these injuries. It all comes down to the first aid you provide and ensuring the black bear is no longer in your vicinity.

Brown Bears

Grizzlies are the most aggressive bear that you will probably encounter. Polar bears are also aggressive, but most of us do not venture into their territory. Kodiak bears are named for an island, Kodiak, in Alaska. They are still brown bears, albeit, they are considered as a separate type since they have been on the island for decades. Brown bears are larger in size, with grizzlies being the largest.

You never want to come between a mom and her cubs, even accidentally. This can be perceived as a threat to the young bears. Males tend to be on their own until it is the mating season or the salmon run.

It can be a great adventure to go out and spot bears when the salmon are swimming and jumping upstream; however, there will be numerous bears along the river, so you never want to go out alone or think that you won't pose a threat if you get close. In fact, you want to choose a river that is near civilization to avoid any dangerous encounters.

Brown bears are found in Glacier, Yellowstone, Denali national parks, the entire state of Alaska, Montana are a few other areas. You definitely want to know if there is any chance of encountering these bears on trails you are going to hike or camp near.

Make sure you do not have food with you or if you are out in the wilderness that you have it packaged appropriately.

Never attempt to kill a bear even if it is attacking you. It is harder to kill them than you think. Even rubber bullets designed to scare them can have the opposite effect.

As with any bear, you do not want to appear as a threat. However, if the bear is intent on attacking, make yourself look as big as possible and make as much noise as you can.

Do not run and do not lose sight of the bear. Like black bears, brown bears can climb, and they are fast.

Brown bears are also larger, which means they can inflict a lot of damage not only with their weight but their claws and teeth. Most bears are going to neutralize the threat and leave. Few will continue attacking. If you can make the bear lose interest and go on their business, that is the best option.

Emergency Care for Brown Bear Attacks

Before you approach an injured party, make sure the bear threat is gone.

1. Begin with calling the person's name and seeing if the individual is responsive. If they are, try to keep the person calm as you assess the injuries and dial emergency numbers.

2. Dial 911 or any other emergency line based on where you are located.

3. Start treating severe injuries, such as significant blood loss. Any arterial bleed or significant blood loss is going to prevent you from saving a person if it is not controlled. The shock will stop the heart.

4. If the person is not breathing and the heart has stopped, your first priority is still to stop any excessive blood loss. CPR will only cause more blood to pump out of the body if there is a large gash or arterial bleed.

5. Once you have applied a tourniquet to any wounds and packed them with gauze to try and stop the bleeding, you can begin CPR.

6. Tilt the head back and raise the chin to straighten the airway. Provide two breaths.

7. Being 100 compressions per minute, pushing as hard and as fast as you can on the person's chest. Done correctly, the ribs will break as you force your hands to press on the heart.

8. Give two more breaths after 100 compressions and continue to repeat the process until the heart starts, breathing starts or help arrives.

9. If the person has not stopped breathing and the heart still pumps, but the person is unconscious, continue checking for wounds and address the primary injuries.

10. You may be told by emergency personnel to remain where you are, or you may be asked to get to a different location to get closer to help.

You want to follow these steps to ensure that you are not going to be hurt. You cannot administer first aid or CPR if you become injured by the bear. Furthermore, you need to dial 911 as soon as possible, even before the attack is over if you can. Sometimes shock can delay our reaction until it is time to take action to help another. Just make sure you dial 911 or whatever number will get emergency personnel to your location as quickly as possible.

Hippos

Unless you intend on traveling to a location where hippopotami live, you should be safe from this deadly animal. But you never know when you might encounter one, such as deciding to become a biologist working at the zoo. Hippos are swift creatures, more so than their size would indicate. They do get on land, but most of their life is spent in the water. They live in rivers or lakes.

A hippo has very sharp teeth, and their bite exudes a significant amount of pressure that can crush a person. You do not want to get in their path. Each year about 500 people die from hippos. In comparison, less than 200 shark attacks occur per year. A hippo's size can also crush a person.

If you are unlucky enough to encounter a hippo in the wild, you want to attack its eyes and avoid being pancaked.

Emergency Care for Hippo Attacks

There are a few scenarios for how a hippo can injure a person: only a bite, being crushed, or both. Depending on the situation, you will need to supply the best emergency care you can until help arrives.

1. Have someone call for help, if possible. It may be faster to get the person to the nearest medical facility rather than waiting for help, given the areas for potential attacks.

2. Make sure the area is clear of hippos before attempting to get to the person.

3. Check the injuries. Is there significant blood loss happening?

4. As with any situation, you need to stop blood loss before you can treat other injuries, even a person without a heartbeat or respiratory response.

5. Use a tourniquet just above the wound if it is a limb. If it is abdominal, you need to pack the wound and wrap bandages as tightly as you can.

6. Once blood loss is stopped, it is time to address any pulse or breathing issues.

7. Remember to tilt the head back to lift the chin and administer breaths in between every 100 to 120 compressions per minute. Push hard and fast.

8. If the heart starts beating and breathing resumes, you can determine the best way to get the person to medical staff.

Tigers

Bengal tigers are known for their deadly attacks, although other tigers can be just as dangerous. There is a true story about an early 1900s attack, thought to be one tiger, that developed a taste for humans. It is said to have killed hundreds of people in less than ten years. Studies have examined the bite marks left by the tiger to confirm it was one and not multiple tigers.

Tigers are large cats that do not like to be threatened or encounter anything they perceive as dangerous. Hungry tigers are even worse because they may stray into human territory rather than staying in the jungle.

Preventing a tiger attack requires staying out of the areas these large cats live. But, if you are going on an adventure, be prepared. Be guided through the area and make sure you remember what to do in an emergency.

Emergency Care

Make sure the tiger is gone.

1. You do not want to reencounter the tiger or, worse, be attacked while attempting to help someone else. Never put

yourself in danger as you will not be able to help the other person.

2. Call for help if you are in an area that has a medical team that can help you.

3. If the person is conscious, try to keep them calm. Shock can set in, and they may become unconscious.

4. Assess the significant injuries first, looking for blood loss.

5. Apply a tourniquet to any limb that shows extreme blood loss. In some instances, loss of limb occurs, so you must get the blood stopped.

6. Check for a pulse, and if they are breathing once, blood loss is controlled.

7. Use CPR, if necessary.

8. Otherwise, get the person to a doctor immediately, while continuing to monitor blood loss and signs of shock that could stop the heart.

Lions

Lions are animals that will attack when hungry and are more likely to eat native African prey, but when food is scarce, you definitely do not want to be in lions hunting path. Hundreds of deaths can be attributed to lions per year for those who live in Africa. As long as you visit and stay with your guide on a safari, you should be safe from an attack. But, being prepared for an incident is helpful should you encounter someone who is not so lucky.

Emergency Protocols

Make sure the lion or lions have left the area before going to help anyone attacked. Call for local help. Sometimes you may need to bring the person to the nearest facility, but you should alert someone you are coming.

1. Get to the injured person.

2. Try to calm the person if they are still conscious.

3. Assess the injuries looking for any wounds that could lead to death by blood loss.

4. Treat the most dangerous wounds first, using a tourniquet or packing the wound with gauze and wrapping bandages around the area.

5. If necessary, restart the heart and get oxygen to the person by using CPR techniques.

6. Get the person to a medical facility, while monitoring for further issues such as shock that could lead to death.

Dogs

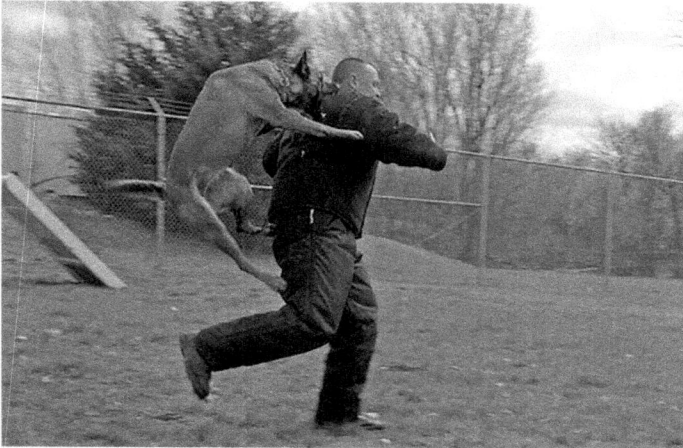

Yes, dogs have made the list, even though we consider them pets and our best friends. Not all dogs are as calm as they appear. Some people even train their dogs to be attack and guard animals. More dog bites happen each year than any of the other animals discussed above. Sometimes a dog does not mean to bite, and other times, it does so because it feels threatened by you. It is essential to get treated for any dog bite that occurs because left untreated; these bites can be life-threatening.

Emergency Care for a Dog Bite

If a dog bites you or someone you are with, you need to provide emergency care.

1. First, flush the wound with alcohol or another cleaning agent from your first aid kit.

2. Wrap the wound.

3. Use ice to help with any swelling caused by the bite.

4. Go to a medical facility. If it takes time to get to a facility, you can take a pain reliever for the swelling and pain. Joint pain is not uncommon with dog bites.

Dog saliva can have any number of bacteria that could cause an infection. You need to get your dog bite treated by a doctor, even if it seems minor.

The physician will ask if you know the dog or if it was an unknown animal. Some dogs can have rabies, just like any other animal. Rabies can kill a person, as well as the dog. So if any animal, including those mentioned in previous chapters, was foaming at the mouth, looking sickly, or feral, you may need treatment for rabies. Caught early, you may survive.

A doctor will clean the wound. They will have a blood test run to see if any infection sets in and then prescribe an antibiotic. If your tetanus is not updated, they will provide a shot. You will monitor the wound to see if it gets worse, including if swelling or extreme pain starts a day or more after the bite.

Domesticated Cats

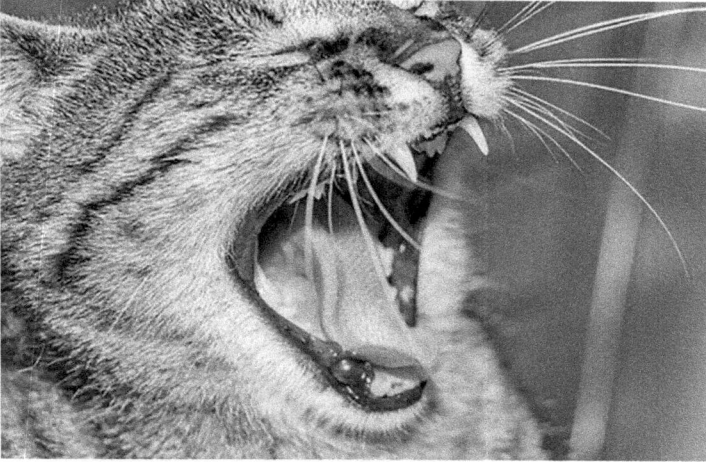

Yes, our household cats can be just as harmful as the large cats out in the wild. Of course, their cute and cuddly appearance doesn't always tell the truth. Accidents and fear can lead to a bite even by our pets. Like dogs, it is an infection that results or rabies that can be life-threatening when a domestic cat bites you.

Sometimes cats get scared in situations or bite during play. Their saliva can contain bacteria that will lead to an infection, usually relating to blood, so it is never wise to treat a wound without a medical professional looking at it.

Emergency Care for a Cat Bite
Begin with first aid.

1. Clean and sanitize the wound.

2. If you are bleeding profusely, which can happen if the animal gets a small artery or vein, make sure you stop the bleeding.

3. Wrap the wound.

4. Apply ice.

5. Take a pain reliever.

6. Get to a medical facility and have the wound checked.

7. The doctor will want to know if you know the animal. If you do not and there is a potential for rabies, they will provide signs and symptoms, plus a protocol for what to do.

8. A blood test will be run to see if there are early signs of infection. Chances are if the wounds are swollen and red, the physician will prescribe an antibiotic. If you are not updated on your tetanus shot, you will get one.

9. You will need to monitor your health and return to the doctor if the wound gets worse or in a week to check the healing progress.

Conclusion

The emergency care you supply is based on the situation, and the danger posed. You always need to make sure the area is clear of danger, whether it is an insect or animal. You do not want someone else to be harmed while attempting to rescue the person attacked.

Insect bites may not be lethal unless an infection sets in, which is why first aid includes keeping the wound clean, dry, and undamaged. You need to wash it and apply an anti-itch cream to stave off any infection. For scorpion stings or more severe reactions, your best method is keeping the heart going and a good supply of oxygen. At the same time, you hurry the injured person to the nearest medical facility.

When it comes to animal bites, blood loss is the number one cause of death. A severed artery can cause a person to bleed out in moments, so it matters less if the heart is beating, and the person is breathing if you cannot stop excessive blood loss.

Remember, to carry this with you as a guide; especially, if you are going into the wilderness and may encounter any number of the animals or insects mentioned.

References

http://www.toxinology.com/fusebox.cfm?fuseaction=main.scorpion
s.results&Common_Names_term=&Family_term=&Genus_
term=Androctonus&Species_term=&countries_terms=&reg
ion_terms=&General_Information__term=

https://www.nationalgeographic.com/animals/invertebrates/group/s
corpions/#:~:text=There%20are%20almost%202%2C000%
20scorpion,against%20that%20species'%20chosen%20prey.

https://www.planetdeadly.com/animals/worlds-dangerous-scorpions

https://www.asgmag.com/prepping/safety-prepping/fatal-stingers-
the-6-deadliest-scorpions-in-the-world/

https://www.medicalnewstoday.com/articles/312484#home_remedi
es_for_fire_ant_stings

https://lakenormanpest.com/top-8-dangerous-ants-time/

https://www.allergy.org.au/patients/insect-allergy-bites-and-
stings/jack-jumper-ant-allergy

https://www.cntraveller.com/gallery/the-10-most-dangerous-
animals-in-the-world

https://www.redcross.org/take-a-class/cpr/performing-cpr/cpr-steps

https://www.britannica.com/list/9-of-the-worlds-deadliest-snakes

https://www.cdc.gov/parasites/sleepingsickness/treatment.html

http://www.walkthroughindia.com/wildlife/top-5-wild-animals-responsible-for-killing-most-humans-in-india/

https://www.bbc.com/news/world-36320744

https://www.floridamuseum.ufl.edu/shark-attacks/yearly-worldwide-summary/

https://www.britannica.com/list/9-of-the-worlds-deadliest-spiders

EMERGENCY CARE

FOR BEGINNERS

How to Handle A Broken Bone

BRANDA NURT

Introduction

E mergency care is essential in any health system because it's the safety net designed to catch and treat critical patients. In 1991, Roemer defined a health system as "the combination of resources, organization, financing, and management that culminate in the delivery of health services to the population." The World Health Organization gave another definition of a health system in 2002: "All activities whose primary purpose is to promote, restore and maintain health."

The critical factor in both definitions is the delivery of health services. Nevertheless, there are things that a non-medical person can do to contribute to the salvage of a persons' health in medical emergencies. Everyone should go to the emergency care department in medical emergencies. Still, some actions or inactions can worsen the situation in the absence of necessary skills such as the means of handling a broken bone. Sometimes, the right kind of treatment, provided as soon as possible, can greatly increase the outcome of the patient's recovery. This makes it important to provide assistance before waiting for the medical professionals to arrive at the scene. In other cases, the medical professionals are unable to reach the scene at all. In these cases, the patients need to be taken to an emergency service by a natural person. Medical professionals can't be everywhere at once, so it's logical to be prepared to fill in whenever they aren't around in an emergency.

Someone who would want to prepare himself to fill in the role of a medical professional in the management of a fracture needs to learn a couple of particular things. This person would need to learn how to identify a possible fracture just by looking at it, limit the damage right there at the scene, prepare the patient to be transferred to a hospital, and even take the patient to a hospital while avoiding further injuries. If you're that kind of person, rest assured that you'll find everything that you need to learn within the pages of this book.

Most fractures can be healed without consequences, particularly fractures in the limbs, which are the most common kinds of fractures. As long as the person receives proper care, the patient should be able to recover full functionality of the affected limb. However, receiving or not receiving proper care can be the difference between a patient with a healed fracture, and a patient who develops a disability due to a fracture.

Mortality as a consequence of fractures is, on the other hand, very uncommon. The only fractured patients in real danger of dying are polytraumatized patients. Patients under these circumstances are the worst case possible, which doesn't mean that we don't have to be ready for these cases. Also, a fractured bone located in a dangerous area can become a life-threatening injury if they're managed in the wrong way. So, in the worst case scenario, the patient will need good treatment to stay alive. In a scenario that's not as serious, the patient could die if he receives the wrong treatment. In any case, your input could be the difference between life and death of these patients.

Fractures can have very serious consequences, and their gruesome and raw nature makes us perceive them as really scary, but they don't need to be. Of course that fractures need to be taken seriously, and it's better to avoid them, but there's nothing to be afraid of if you know how to treat them.

A broken bone isn't a death sentence. It can get very ugly, and if treated the wrong way, it could have awful consequences. If you're one of those people who want to be able to take care of your family in any situations, this is exactly the book for you. Take this knowledge seriously, practice everything that you need to know, and prepare yourself for the odd chance of facing a fractured bone. You may start this book as someone with no medical knowledge at all, but you'll leave this book as someone who's completely able to handle a fracture with confidence.

If you're in a life-threatening or emergency medical situation, seek medical assistance immediately.

Chapter One

The Rationale Behind Emergency Care

When we think about emergency care, our minds usually drift over the picture of an emergency room. Famous TV shows have created an image of emergency care that's much more dramatic than how it goes in the real life. Everything that you'll be applying as fracture treatment is considered emergency care, so it's important to begin by understanding the concept.

Emergency and Life-Threatening Situations

There is an assumption that emergency care is for people who require immediate medical attention because their life is in danger. Amid the urgency, one could take the posture that these people don't choose emergency care because circumstances force them to seek it, but that is not entirely the case. Certain factors are in place, which contributes to the idea that there is a need for emergency care. There is always a compelling incident that needs immediate attention, and this will be illustrated in the following two examples:

1. A person has been involved in an accident, resulting in a broken bone protruding through his skin. Bleeding creates a

need for immediate care because of the excruciating pain, the loss of blood and bone exposure can lead to infection. If the loss of blood is important, this could become a life-threatening situation. However, most fractures aren't life-threatening conditions; that doesn't mean they aren't urgent.

2. The second person is a lady who finds a lump on her breast one morning and has to book an appointment to see a doctor who will establish whether the lump is cancerous. These two people are both experiencing severe medical conditions, but one is more urgent than the other; the broken bone.

In these examples we have a life-threatening situation, which is the possibility of breast cancer. However, cancer treatment isn't acute because this is a chronic illness. Even if this is a disease that could result in death, the treatment could wait until a proper appointment date is set between the doctor and the patient. The first example, on the other hand, isn't in a life-threatening situation. However, this patient's situation needs swift treatment or else there's danger of dire consequences. This is an urgent situation that needs immediate attention or else it could have dangerous consequences.

The Prompt Response and the Right Response in Emergency Care

Emergency care situations require someone who has knowledge and skill to address it, which isn't available to everyone. Emergency care situations pertain to medical matters, and anyone attempting to resolve the medical emergency without medical knowledge could further harm the victim. An example would be in cases of a fractured bone. A person can attempt to move someone who has stated that they are in extreme pain, but if a section of their limb has changed color, he's unable to move it, and there is swelling, there is probably a fracture. Attempting to move this patient without immobilizing the limb could deteriorate the situation of the fracture, harming the patient, and worsening his chances at recovery. So, as harsh as this reality may seem, it's better to wait for someone who knows how to treat a fractured patient than to try to help the patient without the required knowledge.

In emergency care, the treatment of a patient should arrive as soon as possible. However, if the help comes from a person without knowledge or training, sometimes it's better not to receive prompt treatment at all. If you don't know how to prepare a patient for transportation to a hospital, then it's better to wait for a trained paramedic to pick up the patient and take him for specialized medical attention. Prompt attention is extremely important, but that doesn't mean that you should try to give it under any circumstances. In the particular case of fractured bones, making the situation worse is so easy that it's better to leave these injuries be if you don't know how to treat them. This is the nature of the emergency care. Even if it requires a swift response, this response isn't an obligation for everyone around the injured patient. Sometimes, the best choice you can make is to ask for help and wait for the help to arrive.

If you're in a life-threatening or emergency medical situation, seek medical assistance immediately.

Chapter Two

Anatomic Considerations
Regarding Bones

There are several complex processes happening at once during the embryologic development of a human being. Bone tissue, like any other tissue in the human body, is created through the interactions and evolution of cells in the embryo.

Anatomy of the Human Body

There's a particular language used to describe the anatomy of the human body. This language assumes the heart as the point of reference, being seen as the center of the body. One should picture the body in the standing up position, facing ahead with arms raised and the hands facing forward. With this anatomical position as a basic point of reference, the rest of the terms used in the description of anatomy take meaning. The different terms used for anatomical reference, the same ones used as a reference for fractures, are the following:

Proximal and distal

Proximal refers to the area that is near the heart, while distal is further from the heart. An example of this would be that the shoulder is proximal to the elbow while the elbow is distal from the shoulder.

Anterior and posterior

Anterior refers to the front part of the human body while the posterior refers to the back. An example would the breasts being anterior to the sternum, while the back is posterior to the lungs.

Medial and lateral

Medial refers to the middle part of the body, while lateral is the body's outer area. An example would be the nose is medial to the ears while the ears are lateral to the lips.

Location of fractures

Once that we have this knowledge in mind, we can use it to describe fractures. A fracture can be distal to the elbow if it's in the wrist, or it can be proximal to the knee if it's in the femur. These terms are universal, so they can be used to describe injuries to any medical professional without fear of being misunderstood.

Bones of a Human Being

The skeletal system is union of the different bones, cartilage, and joints within the body. Its main function is to act as a support frame for the rest of the body tissues. Muscles are directly attached to the bones through the tendons, and the rest of the organs are held within and around the skeletal system. Also, the skeletal system allows us to move, as muscle wouldn't be able to create motion without the pivotal structures they act upon. Also, the skeletal system allows us to stand against gravity, essential for movement. The next main function of the skeletal system is to provide protection to the vulnerable organs. The ribcage, for example, is there to protect the lungs and the heart. This makes a fractured rib a particularly dangerous fracture, since it could compromise the integrity of the organs held within them. The next functions, more important for life sustenance in the long term, are blood cells production and the storage of minerals. If any part of the frame that gets broken, i.e., fractured, this affects every single one of these functions. The affected body segment will lose its shape, it won't be able to move properly, and the contiguous structures of the body will be in danger, if not directly affected by the fracture.

You could start your study of the skeletal system by taking a look at all the bones pictures below.

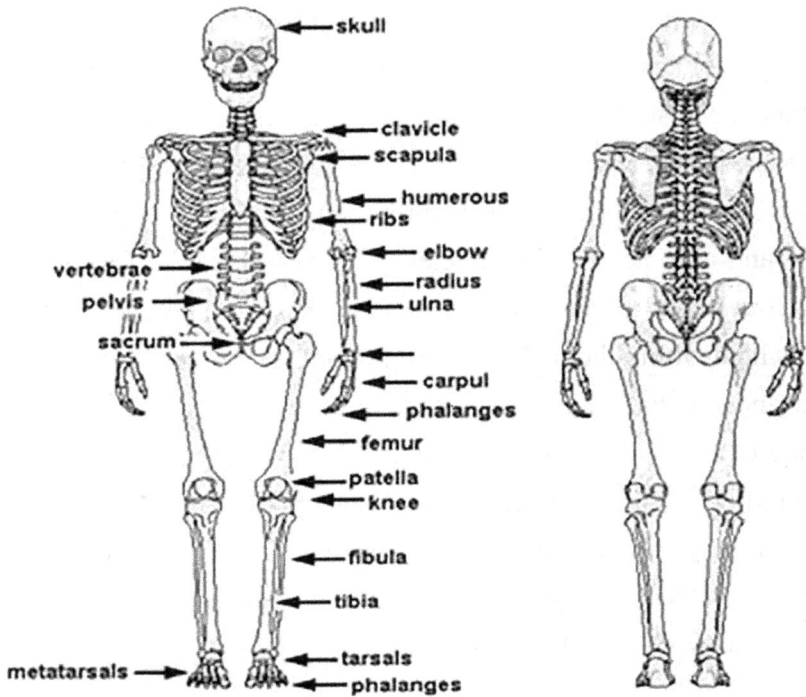

Each bone stands as an individual organ; for example, the femur or the ribs are all single organs. These different organs, collectively, form the skeleton. The skeleton is the only organ system that is preserved for many years through fossilization. This preservation nature is the only way that humans have been able to establish the evolution of other living organisms and even extinct animals. The tissue characteristic of a bone allows for its conservation as a fossil for years, thus preserving the history and allowing further studies.

Types of Bones

Bones in the human body are different, however, they can be classified in different types according to their morphological qualities. The types of bones present in the body are the following:

Long bones

These bones can be described as having a long and tubular shape. They range from the femur to the small phalanges in the hands. They're mostly found in the limbs, and their main function is to facilitate movement. Even if they're strong, since they're part of the limbs, long bones are frequently fractured. The metaphysis, a particularly weak part of the strong bones is where most of these fractures happen.

Flat bones

Flat bones can take a long shape, such as the ribs, or they can take a wide shape, such as the bones of the skull. Their main morphological quality is that they're not tubular, but flat. Their main function is to act like a shield and protect the organs of the body. Their shapes allow them to be very strong, so it's uncommon for them to be fractured. So, hip fractures (the strongest flat bones in the body) are only common among people with underlying diseases, such as osteoporosis.

Short bones

These bones can be described to have the shape of a dice. They often take the shape of an irregular cube, and they're present in the joints of the wrist and the ankle. These can be fractured, and such fractures are harder to identify because they often don't cause deformation. Which is the reason why any injury produced by blunt force applied to these areas should be considered a fracture, and the affected limb should be immobilized.

Sesamoid bones

Sesamoid bones are small, round, flat, and they always go in the tendons. These are more often dislocated than fractured, since any damaging force applied to them will rather take them outside of their anatomical place instead of breaking them. The patella, the small bone in front of the knee joint, is a sesamoid bone.

Irregular bones

These are bones with extravagant shapes that can't fit in any of the other categories. Their shape allows them to fulfill multiple functions while also providing protection to the structures inside the body. The vertebra are an example of irregular bones. Its shape protects the spinal cord while allowing blood vessels, nerves, and muscles to attack to it in different specialized places.

Parts of a Bone

Learning about the different parts of a bone will teach us where to look when we're assessing a fracture. It will also teach us what to expect to find in a broken bone, and how do the bones work in general.

Diaphysis

The diaphysis is the tubular part of the long bone. It's long, regular, and strong, so it can withstand a lot of damage and stress before breaking. It's uncommon to find a broken diaphysis, so you shouldn't start looking at the middle of the limbs for a possible fracture. Long bones will only be broken in the diaphysis if extreme force is applied directly to it.

Epiphysis

If the diaphysis is the shaft of the long bone, the epiphysis can be described as the two ends of the shaft. Purposed as the place where the different bones are jointed together, epiphysis have different shapes, but they're also very strong. A fractured epiphysis is uncommon since any blunt force applied in the joint of the limbs will more likely dislocate the joint instead of breaking the bone. However, long bones can still be broken in the epiphysis if there's an underlying disease making that part of the bone weaker, or if very violent force is applied directly to it.

Metaphysis

This is the small place between the diaphysis and each epiphysis of any long bone. In growing humans, the metaphysis will be the place in which the tissue formation and growing happens. Because of this, the metaphysis is the weakest part of the long bones, and exactly where you should look when assessing a possible fracture. Even in adults, metaphysis are still the weakest part of the broken bones.

Compact bone

This is the strongest tissue of the bone. In long bones, there's compact bone following the shape of the whole bone, creating a hollow structure similar to a tube that's filled with either spongy bone or bone marrow. In flat bones, there are two layers of compact bone around one layer of spongy bone. So, if the outer layer of the flat bone were to be broken (in the skull, for example), the inner layer of compact bone should still be able to protect the brain.

Compact bone is strong and reliable, but it can be dangerous. When it's completely broken, the pieces of compact bone can be sharp and harmful, which is the reason why moving a fractured patient in the wrong way could become a life-threatening situation. The edges of broken compact bone are capable of cutting muscular tissue, nerves, and even blood vessels.

Compact bone tissue is mostly formed of extracellular matrix, which is very rich in minerals, so it's the specialized tissue in the bones that fulfills the function of mineral storage.

Medullary cavity

This is the space located within the diaphysis of the long bones. It's function is to give space to the bone marrow. It shouldn't be confused with the spinal canal, which is the space within the vertebra that holds the spinal cord.

Spongy bone

Softer tissue of the bone, usually present in the epiphysis of the long bones and inside the rest of the bones. It's very porous, vascularized, and softer than compact bone. Spongy bone is mostly formed of cells, it doesn't have as much extracellular matrix as the compact bone, so it's not a strong.

Periosteum

The periosteum is a thin layer that covers the bones. All muscle and tendon insertions happen in the periosteum, it also carries the blood vessels and the nerves of the bones. Apart from providing sustenance to the bones, the periosteum works as a barrier to protect fractures and deformation in the bones. This role is more important in children, where the periosteum is stronger than ever, avoiding full fractures of the bones and creating what's known as greenstick fractures (fractures in which only one side of the periosteum and compact bone is broken).

Endosteum

It's a thin layer that covers the medullary cavity; it's highly vascularized, so it provides nutrition to the inner tissue of the long bones.

Bone Marrow

This is specialized soft tissue found within the spongy bone of all bones, and the medullary cavity of the long bones. It can be divided in red bone marrow and yellow bone marrow.

Red bone marrow is the tissue specialized for blood-cell production. It's the only kind of bone marrow that we have as children, until we start to grow up and the red bone marrow present inside the medullary cavity is slowly replaced by the yellow bone marrow.

The yellow bone marrow, on the other hand, is the type of bone tissue specialized in fat storage. Once we're adults, yellow bone marrow is the only type of bone marrow present in the medullary cavity. So, red bone marrow is mainly found in hip bones, ribs, vertebra, and sternum.

Bone Formation and Collagen

The tissue component in bone consists of specialized cells and an extracellular matrix that is full of minerals. 70% of the extracellular matrix of the bone is organically composed of a fibrous protein called collagen. Different forms of collagen can even be found in other body tissues.

Various types of collagen can be found in the body, but only ten have been identified. These ten types of collagen are named using the numbers from class I to X. The collagen found in bones is type I collagen, which is also a component in connective tissues such as teeth, tendons, ligaments, and skin.

Cartilage is a connective tissue in the human body that can be found on the outer surface of bones, as well as in the joints between bones. Cartilage is composed of type II collagen, which is the main component of collagen, therefore identifying it as cartilage-type collagen.

Early in its development, bone exists as osteoid, an organic, unmineralized matrix surrounding the bone cells which deposited it. The next phase of bone formation is the mineralization of this extracellular matrix through the deposition of calcium phosphate.

This allows the bones to fossilize. This stage of mineral deposition is crucial because it is what has led to the modern-day identification of bones by isolating phosphoproteins. The phosphorous proteins are usually osteonectin and osteocalcin, and they take up 1 to 5% of the bone matrix, but it should be noted that these minerals only appear within the bone matrix after mineralization and not in the beginning stage of specialization of bone cells.

There are two main paths for bone formation, direct development and substitution of another tissue. These two means of formation of bones undergo different forms of inductive interactions.

Substitution of Another Tissue

Bones can be formed from the replacement of tissue such as cartilage, which leads to the creation of the long bones (limbs), vertebra, and ribs. These bones are therefore referred to as replacement bones. Replacement bones bring the question as to the origin of cartilage. It has been researched the formation of cartilage from the embryo stage to the point of being replaced by bone tissue.

It has been reported that there must be external factors that will influence the formation of cartilage within the body at the cellular level. Thus, there is no self-distinction in the creation of cartilage cells, but instead, there must be inductive interaction. An example of possible inductive interaction would be that the cells in the face need to interact with the epithelia so that they can lead to specialization and form cartilage cells. Some studies propose that the cartilage cells mutate on their own to form bone cells and bone tissue; another possibility is that, as the cells of the cartilage die naturally, the cells surrounding the cartilage change into bone cells and bone tissue.

At the cartilage stage, before being replaced by bone tissue, there's a cellular membrane that borders the cartilage known as the perichondrium. This is the same membrane that later surrounds the bone, turning into the periosteum. It's clear that the perichondrium transitions to the periosteum after the cartilage is replaced by bone. The transformation of perichondrium to periosteum is crucial, if this transformation doesn't take place, it can lead to conditions such as dwarfism.

There is speculation that bone cells are originated in another part of the body and delivered through the blood supply to the cartilage for bone formation. The cartilage matrix is then broken down through the transportation of the bone cells in the blood vessels. Therefore, the movement of the bone cells in the blood vessels is essential for the formation of bones.

Direct Development

The bones of the skull and the clavicle are bones that are not formed through the replacement of cartilage with bone cells. These bones are created through direct development, which is another path for bone formation. These bones are formed inside a membrane of connective tissue, thus giving them the name of membrane bones.

At the embryonic stage of human development, there is much movement that occurs at a cellular level that will result in the development of membrane bones. This movement tends to last days to weeks before the formation of a bone begins. It is worth noting that the creation of the membrane bones of the facial skeleton and the skull takes place in the early stages, making them very crucial in the structure of the nervous system.

Chapter Three

Fractures and Identifying Fractures

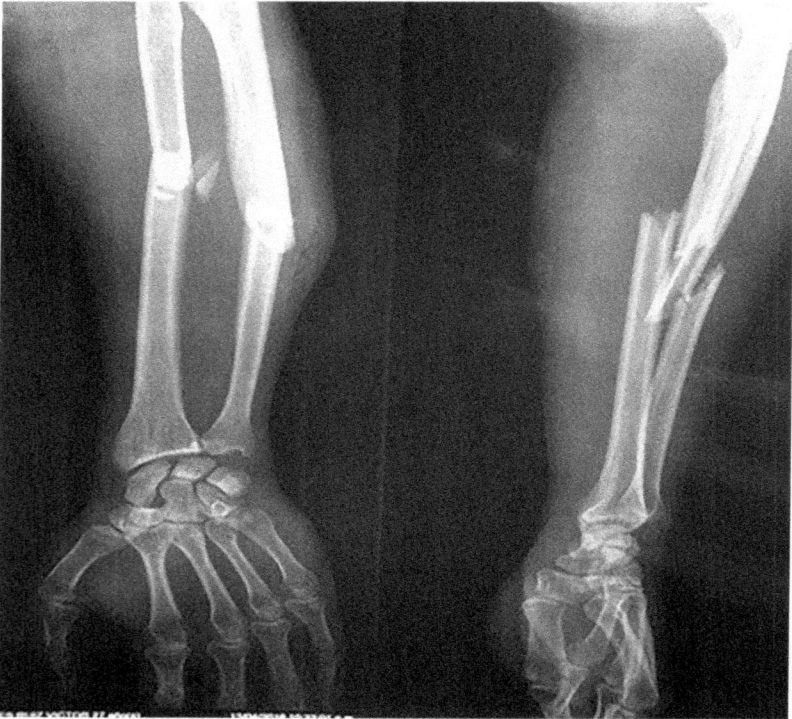

In this picture you may see that the radius and the ulna are split in half. You may guess that, since they're split in the diaphysis, this patient's forearm must have endured a huge amount of stress. Later in this book we'll see how to call this specifically, but right now all we can say is that this is a fracture. A fracture can be defined as the broken continuity of a bone. This means that the bone has either been partially or completely broken. The bone can either have a small crack, or break into two or more pieces. The treatment of the fractured bone depends on the location of the fracture and the level of deformation.

Fractures do not usually result in the death of the victim, but some other factors could be life-threatening, such as the infection of the open wound and the rupture of important blood vessels. Despite this fact, fractures aren't usually deadly; however, they must be immediately addressed because they are extremely painful, and failure to quickly address them could result in external pressure being exerted to that area, thus worsening the fracture. During emergency care of broken bones, one needs to be very careful because the wrong move could deteriorate the situation and worsen the fracture. This is the reason why it's so important to learn how to treat a fracture correctly.

Identifying a Fractured Bone

It's one thing to see someone who fell from a tree and believe that he may have a fractured bone, and it's an entirely different matter to be able to recognize the signs and symptoms of a fracture. Identifying a fracture is the first step before attempting to treat it, so it's important that you learn the symptoms and signs of a fractured bone.

Swelling or bruising

The affected area of the fracture will always exhibit swelling, and sometimes even bruising. Swelling will be present because a fracture is always a traumatic event, so the body will answer with an inflammatory reaction, producing and increase in volume in the affected area, as well as a reddish taint in the skin.

The bruising will be present if there's bleeding around the fracture, which will almost always be the case. As we've learned in the previous chapter, bones have vascular irrigation in the periosteum, so a fractured bone will bleed through its broken blood vessels. Also, the same traumatic energy that fractured the bone could've broken the muscular or vascular tissue around it, producing the bleeding and bruising. In some cases, the edges of the pieces of the fractured bone could damage the surrounding blood vessels. If this last scenario happens with a fractured femur, breaking the femoral artery, as an example of a bone damaging a large blood vessel, the fracture becomes a life-threatening incident.

Deformity

The fractured area of the bony may lose its natural morphological characteristics. A fractured forearm may be bent in ways that aren't natural, for example. This isn't always the case, and fractures without deformity are far better for the patient than those in which the affected area loses its natural form. However, deformity is possible, and it's a very clear sign of a fracture.

Pain

A fracture is almost always extremely painful. The victim will scream in pain, pointing to the affected area. This happens because the bone, an organ of the body with nerves and sensitivity, has been traumatized, and it gets worse every time the patient tries to move the affected area. Another reason behind the pain is that muscles and tendons contract around the fractured bone. Further examination can't be done because manipulating the affected area will increase the pain.

Loss of functionality

A fractured area can't move normally, in most cases it can't move at all. Bones are a fundamental pillar of the process of locomotion, so a broken bone will render the muscles attached to it unable to create movements. Also, in most cases, the patient won't be able to tolerate any weight over the affected area, so the patient won't be able to step over a fractured foot, for example.

Open fracture

There's a particular kind of fracture that can be identified as soon as you see the patient, and it's the open fracture. In this case, a segment of the broken bone has pierced the skin and it can be seen protruding through the skin. In these cases, there's no need to look for the rest of the signs to identify and diagnose the fracture; however, in these cases the patient must be taken with greater urgency to a hospital.

Some Exceptions to the Rule

The previous signs and symptoms are present in almost every fracture, and those are the ones you should be looking for when you try to identify a fracture. However, in some cases, you could find a fracture that follows a completely different path.

Some fractures are painless, and even show lack of sensitivity. This is because the injury caused nerve damage, so the patient is unable to feel pain. In some cases, the patient is unable to feel even simple touch. This is atypical, but it's also a situation that should turn on your alarms and make you think that there's something wrong with the patient. Fractures usually happen after severe trauma, so it shouldn't be normal to fall from a tree over your arm and not feel any pain in the affected arm.

Some patients are able to move their fractures, and even put weight over them. This happens because the fracture didn't abandon its anatomical position, and the tendons and muscle around the fractured bone are working to keep everything in place. The person may be able to move the affected area, but the pain and swelling will still be there, and they will be intense.

Swelling and bruises are the usual signs of a fracture, but sometimes the skin's color goes the other way and it turns pale instead. This happens because there has been an interruption of the blood flow way over the affected area.

Looking for the obvious

Fractures are almost always caused by trauma, so you'll only look for them in an injured patient. Car accidents, falls, sports accidents, fights, these are all situations in which you should consider the possibility of a fractured bone. As we'll see later in this book, sometimes fractures aren't caused by intense trauma. In these cases, you'll still see the signs and symptoms of a fracture, you'll just have to think about the possibility and look for it.

Applying the knowledge

Fractures are very delicate injuries that must be handled carefully. As we'll see later when we study the treatment and management of a fracture, you should avoid movements and efforts by all means. So, even if the loss of functionality is a sign of a fracture, making the patient put his weight over his foot to make sure it's fractured is a terrible idea. You should learn how to identify it, and use the information during the interrogation of the patient. You don't need to see the patient trying to take a step with his injured foot to diagnose the fracture, all you need is to ask the patient whether he was able to step over his foot or not before you arrived.

Take the knowledge and use it to ask the right questions. Never compromise the health and recovery of the patient. If you're not entirely sure if what you have in front of you is a fracture or not, you should always think about a fracture first and treat it that way. It's better to be mistaken and immobilize a limb that didn't need to be immobilized than to move a limb that was fractured and increase the injury because you weren't sure about your diagnosis.

If you're in a life-threatening or emergency medical situation, seek medical assistance immediately.

Chapter Four

Types and Causes of Fractures

Fractures are caused by many reasons, but the main thing that must occur is significant external pressure being exerted on a bone, thus leading to a break or cracking of the affected bone. The amount of force needed to fracture a bone depends on the location of the harming force, the bone affected, where it's affected, and the overall health of the bone and the patient. You'll need to understand the usual causes of a fracture to help you diagnose and manage fractures in patients. The leading causes of fractures can be categorized into three, which are traumatic fractures, stress fractures, and pathological fractures.

Traumatic Fractures

These are, by far, the most common types of fractures. The patient suffers a traumatic event that applies enough force to a bone to be able to break it. These fractures can be really dangerous depending on the affected area, since the same force that was able to fracture a bone could also have harmed the organs behind it, so these patients have additional reasons to get medical assessment and treatment as soon as possible.

Traumatic fractures can be divided between direct and indirect fractures.

Direct Fractures

Considered the most violent fractures, direct fractures are those in which the force that causes them is directly applied over them. These fractures are often caused by violent force applied to the body, such as the blast of an explosion, a weapon, or a heavy object falling directly over the bone. They always occur right where the traumatic force is applied.

Indirect Fractures

These traumatic fractures occur in a different place from the application of force. They're an indirect result of pressure, weight, or stress applied elsewhere. They can be avulsion fractures, compression fractures, rotation fractures, or flexion fractures.

Avulsion fractures are similar to stress fractures, and they can be thought of as the ultimate consequence of these types of fractures. Avulsion fractures happen when a tendon or a muscle inserted over a bone exerts so much force over it that it breaks it, causing a fracture. Just like stress fractures, avulsion fractures are mostly common in athletes, particularly in high-performance athletes such as weight-lifters.

Compression fractures happen only in spongy bone. These kinds of fractures are a result of the compression of a segment of the bone between two bones due strong force, pressure, or weight translated to that bone. In the example of someone who falls from a long distance and lands over his feet, the fall could directly fracture the bones in his feet, and indirectly fracture his lower vertebra by compression.

Rotation fractures occur mainly in long bones that are violently rotated, creating a spiral fracture. An example of this would be a person spinning over one of his legs with his foot flat over the floor. The strong of this rotation may be enough to fracture the bone.

Flexion fractures are those where the body of the patient experiences a violent and often abnormal flexion that's able to fracture the bones involved. For example, any form of violent flexion is able to fracture the affected vertebra. The sternum could be fractured by a violent flexion of the thoracic spine (as well as the vertebra at the middle of the thoracic spine).

Stress Fractures

Stress fractures are also caused by strength and pressure applied to the bone. However, in this case, instead of a traumatic and sudden amount of stress applied during an accident or another critical situation, the bone is harmed by the repetitive stress applied by the muscles until it ultimately gives in and breaks.

Stress fractures are only common in endurance athletes, mostly athletes that spend too much time running such as marathonists. Since the bones in the body that are under the largest amount of weight and pressure are the bones of the legs, the legs and the feet will be the preferred place for stress fractures.

Stress fractures usually start as incomplete fractures. The bone will exhibit small cracks that will only be noticeable by using advanced image exploration such as radiographies. These small cracks are called hairline fractures, and it's the most common way in which a stress fracture will present itself. The patient will experience pain and swelling that will get worse with the exercise. This situation will deteriorate until the underlying issue is identified and the patient is treated with immobilizations and rest.

This type of fracture usually isn't the one you'll find in an emergency, but a stress fracture can deteriorate until it goes from a crack in the bone to a complete rupture in the bone (with an avulsion fracture, for example), so it's important to be prepared for it.

Pathological Fracture

There are medical conditions that cause bones to be naturally weak, making these bones prone to fractures, even with minimal force applied. The knowledge of pathological fractures is useful if you're assessing a patient with a fracture that has no reason to be. A pathological fracture can happen because of everyday activities such as bending over and stepping off a car, so fractures don't always need severe trauma or intense physical activity. All you need to know is whether the patient is a healthy patient or not, and for that, you need to conduct a survey on the patient. With this knowledge, and understanding the signs and symptoms to identify and diagnose a fracture, you'll be able to recognize and treat a patient with a pathological fracture. The following medical conditions are the most common causes of a pathological fracture.

Bone Cancer

This is one of the most common causes of a pathological fracture. A bone tumor has a high capacity to weaken the affected bone because it replaces the bone cells and the compact bone tissue with vulnerable tissue. This means that every time you suspect a pathological fracture, you must ask the patient about whether he suffers or has a history of cancer. It doesn't need to be bone cancer; any kind of cancer, especially cancer in the connective tissue such as skin cancer, can become bone cancer through metastasis.

Osteomyelitis

Osteomyelitis is a deep infection of the bone tissue, and it can weaken the structure of the bone to the point it leaves it vulnerable to pathological fractures. Osteomyelitis usually starts as a skin infection that then travels to the underlying bone, so a history of skin or soft-tissue infections around the fractured are will tell you what you need to know about the diagnosis of a pathological fracture.

Osteoporosis and Osteomalacia

Both of these medical conditions weaken the structure of the bones, due to a lack of either calcium or vitamin D. Some patients will already know that they're suffering from these conditions, but if they don't, you should suspect any of these medical conditions in patients of old age and poor diets who often complain about muscle soreness.

Pharmacological Causes

Drugs, albeit an uncommon cause for a pathological fracture, should be considered when there's nothing else. Cancer treatment, blood-pressure treatment, and steroids are examples of pharmacological treatments that are able to weaken the bones.

Other Causes

There are some medical conditions that are rare, difficult to diagnose, and able to produce a pathological fracture. Osteogenesis imperfecta, for example, is a genetic disease where the affected bone has been formed incorrectly, leading to weak bone that could be easily fractured. These are impossible to identify without a professional physician and medical equipment, so the only value they provide to the process of diagnosing a pathological fracture is knowing that, sometimes, the cause can't be identified in a prehospital environment.

Combined Causes

These two main types of fractures, the stress and pathological fractures, are considered apart from the traumatic fractures. However, their force mechanisms may be similar, if considerably lower. A stress fracture can become an avulsion fracture, flexion fracture, or rotation fracture under the right circumstances. The force needed to turn a stress fracture to an avulsion fracture is just lower than the force needed to produce any of these traumatic fractures in a healthy bone.

In the case of pathological fractures, there's always some sort of traumatic force behind them. A patient with a severe underlying disease, such as bone cancer, can experience a hip fracture after sneezing too hard; that doesn't mean it's not also an avulsion fracture, for example, it's just an avulsion fracture in a bone that has been severely weakened by a disease, and therefore, the amount of strength needed to break the bone was minimal.

It's important to understand the mechanisms behind a fracture before attempting to identify them. Once you learn this knowledge, the process of identifying and treating a fracture becomes possible.

If you're in a life-threatening or emergency medical situation, seek medical assistance immediately.

Chapter Five

Common Broken Bones

There are bones in the human body that are more prone to fractures than others, and they include:

- Collarbone

- Forearm

- Ankle

- Wrist

- Hips

- Legs

- Hands and Fingers

Open fractures are much less common than closed fractures. Children usually experience more fractures on their arms, particularly on the metaphysis of the radius and the ulna.

Broken Hands and Fingers

Humans use their fingers and hands a lot during their daily activities, for writing, texting, carrying items, and so on. These constant actions cause fractures to occur a lot in this region. The doctor must ensure that there is no damage to the tendons or nerve as a result of the fracture. Damage to these areas affects the functionality of the hand and fingers. Procedures involving these fractures are very complicated, and specialized surgeons are often involved. The thumb and hands are full of tendons and nerves which facilitate the specialized movements of these parts. The expectation of the healing standards of the arm and legs are not the same as the hand. Treatment of these kinds of fractures is done using a cast or splint, and, in most cases, surgery may be needed.

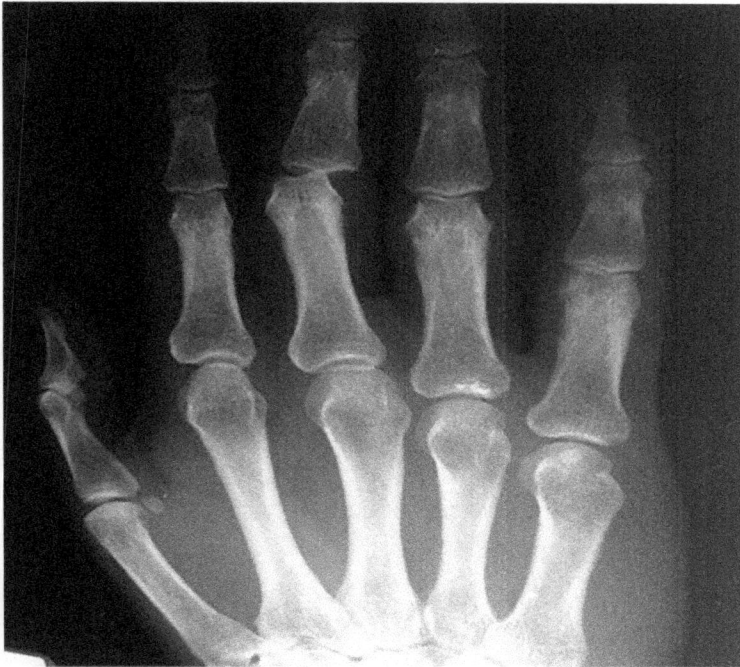

Fractured Wrist

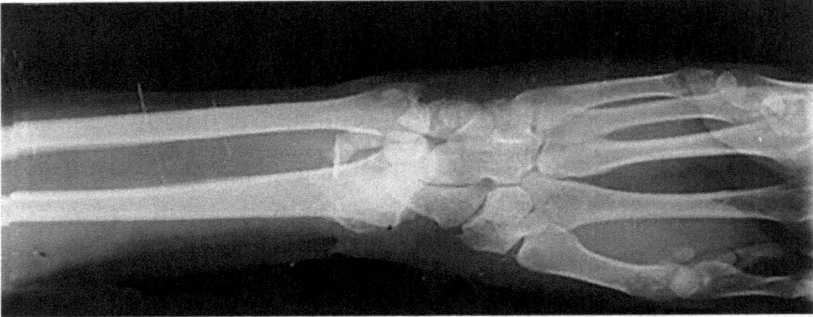

Most wrist fractures occur as a result of falling over the hand. In most cases, the breach on the wrist is associated with another bone. One of the bones that tend to be associated with the wrist bone is the phalanges. Most of these fractures occur in the metaphysis of the radius and the ulna.

The problem with this kind of fracture is that there could be hidden fractures that could even be missed during a radiographic examination because of its positioning and the fact there may be a small fracture that is very difficult to see.

This kind of fracture may or may not need surgery. It would depend on the severity of the injury and the alignment of the bone. The bones of the wrist must be aligned because failure could result in arthritis later on in life. Also, an optimal structure of the wrist is needed for all the range of the hand's movements. So, if the bones can't be properly aligned with medical reduction, surgery is always needed.

Fractured Hip

Fractures located in this region are prevalent amongst the elderly, particularly those who are more than 75 years old. Osteoporosis is one of the significant causes of hip fractures, other than that there are causes such as trauma and falling accidents.

Most hip fractures need surgery, they're extremely painful fractures, and they tend to create disability in the patient.

Fractured Leg

Most of the bones that are at the lower region of the body stand at a high risk of breaking. The leg fractures also include the knee joint, and the type of treatment will depend on the severity of the breach. There are some cases where total knee replacement is necessary because of the severe nature of the fracture.

Other fractures occur on the ankle as well. It is also important to note that fractures on a foot are just as complicated as those that occur on the hand. The reason for this issue is that the diagnostics process is challenging to establish on a radiography.

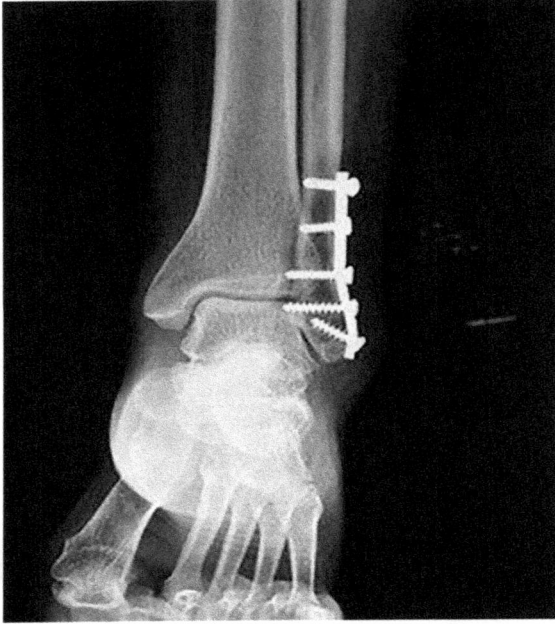

Fractured Toe

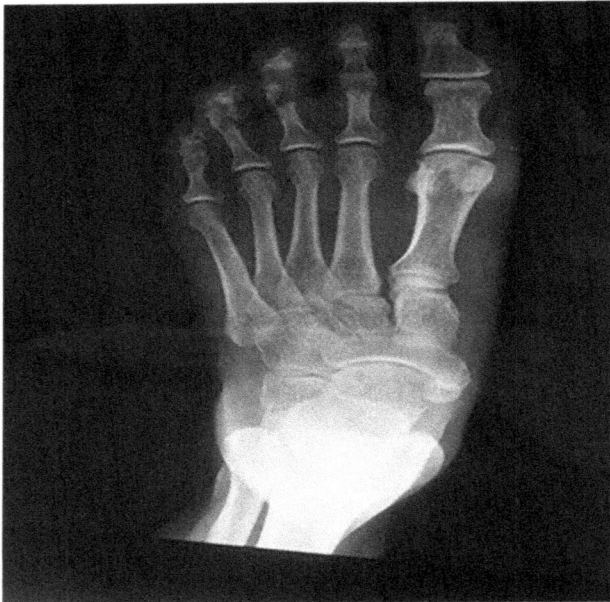

These kinds of fractures are prevalent. They're examined physically, for example, through a pain range test. There are situations where a radiography is the only way to identify this fracture, which is a common stress fracture, but in some cases the fracture can be identified only through the clinic of the patient.

Broken Shoulder

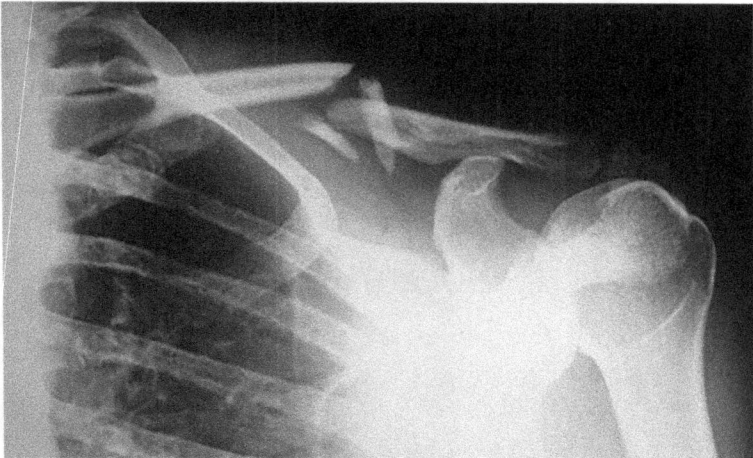

The collarbone fracture is prevalent in all age groups. The elderly tends to get this fracture from falling, while it's more often caused by trauma arising from road accidents and sports injuries in younger people.

Surgery will depend on the number of fractures that have occurred within the shoulder. If the fracture isn't too complicated or severe, treatment is usually done using a sling.

Unlike the collarbone, the shoulder blade is much less likely to fracture. This usually only happens when a great deal of pressure is exerted over the shoulder blade. A shoulder blade fracture is not examined on its own because it usually accompanies other injuries.

Rib Fractures

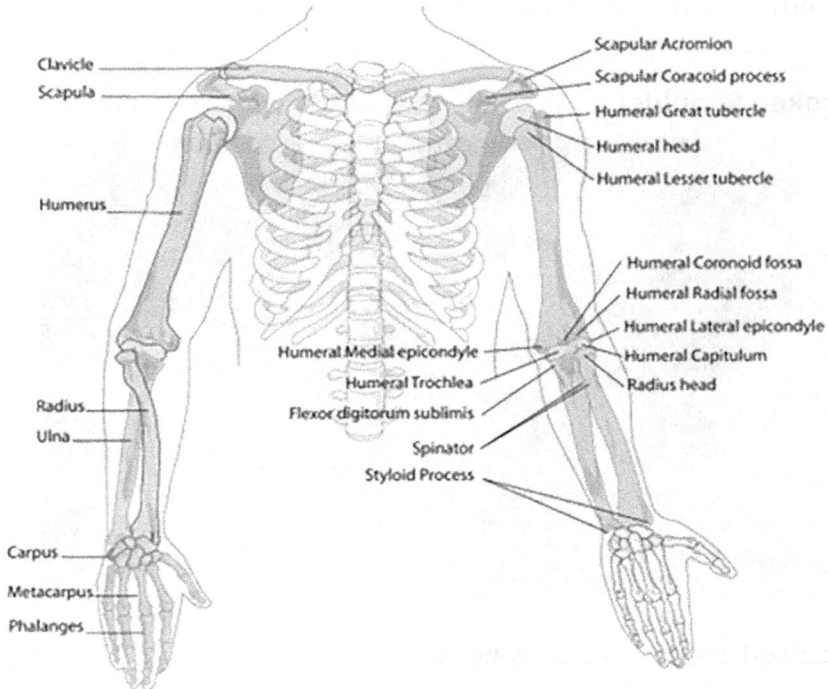

Labels (left side): Clavicle, Scapula, Humerus, Radius, Ulna, Carpus, Metacarpus, Phalanges

Labels (right side): Scapular Acromion, Scapular Coracoid process, Humeral Great tubercle, Humeral head, Humeral Lesser tubercle, Humeral Coronoid fossa, Humeral Radial fossa, Humeral Lateral epicondyle, Humeral Capitulum, Radius head

Labels (center): Humeral Medial epicondyle, Humeral Trochlea, Flexor digitorum sublimis, Spinator, Styloid Process

Rib fractures are only common because of sport and car accidents. The treatment process of rib fractures is different from other areas in the body because they protect organs such as the heart.

It would be essential to note that fractures on the ribs are only treated through pain management. The rationale behind this is to give room for the lungs to expand and contract during the inhalation and exhalation process. Unlike other fractures, rib fractures are not wrapped or bandaged because that will hinder their movement during breathing, which could be very dangerous to a patient. Rib fractures usually heal between 4 to 6 weeks in which the patient will suffer a lot of pain.

If you're in a life-threatening or emergency medical situation, seek medical assistance immediately.

Chapter Six

Classification of Fractures

Fractures are usually set out based on the location of the breach, the bone alignment, and the state of the skin after the injury. This form of description of fractures aids medical personnel identify the specific fracture that is being referred to. Fractures are classified as open or closed fractures, their displacement, the trace, as well as other specific types of fractures. The most important types of fractures to understand in a clinical prehospital setting are the open, closed, displaced, and non-displaced fractures.

Open and Closed Fractures

This classification of fractures is easy to assess and diagnose by anyone with the required knowledge, without needing a radiography or any other types of medical equipment. Open fractures are those in which the bone is in direct contact with the surface, and closed fractures are those in which the bone isn't in direct contact with the body. This means that the bone has pierced through the skin in open fractures, while it remains under the skin in closed fractures.

Open fractures are much more dangerous than closed fractures, as the patient is exposed to infections and the force that took the bone fragment through the skin may have also harmed a blood vessel. Closed fractures, on the other hand, aren't as dangerous as open fractures. They're slightly harder to diagnose, but the patient has a better chance at recovery.

Displaced and Non-Displaced

Broken bones can be displaced or not, and this depends on the bone's alignment after the fracture. A fracture that loses its anatomical form is a displaced fracture, while a fracture that remains in its usual anatomical form is a non-displaced fracture.

Displaced fractures are much easier to identify than non-displaced fractures, and they're also far more dangerous. The edges of a displaced fracture could damage the structures surrounding the affected bone. These are the fractures in which the affected segment will lose its shape. Non-displaced fractures are less dangerous, as well as much harder to diagnose. Some medical professionals have stated that all breaches have a form of displacement and state that the actual term should be 'minimal' displacement rather than non-displacement. However, the terms used are still displaced and non-displaced fractures, and these can usually be identified clinically.

Complete and Incomplete Fractures

Sometimes a fracture won't break the affected bone completely. If the trace of the fracture doesn't reach the whole circumference of the bone, this is an incomplete fracture. If, on the other hand, the trace of the fracture affects the whole bone, it's a complete fracture. Complete fractures are those were the trace affects the whole bone. These distinctions can only be made by a clinician as long as they're within non-displaced fractures. Displaced fractures can almost always be differentiated from incomplete fractures, unless the incomplete fracture is a greenstick fracture, which can also be displaced.

Diaphyseal Fractures

As their name infers, diaphyseal fractures are located in the diaphysis of the long bones. They're classified in simple fractures, complex fractures, and multiple fractures, depending on the trace of the rupture in the bone. These distinctions can only be made by a physician with the help of a radiology.

Simple Fractures

In these fractures, both fragments of the bone are in contact during the complete trace of the fracture. They can be spiral fractures, transversal fractures, and oblique fractures depending on the angle and the shape of their trace.

Complex Fractures

The two main fragments of the bone are in contact in at least one point of the trace of the fracture. They're more dangerous than simple fractures.

Comminuted Fractures

Also called multiple fractures, the comminuted fractures are those in which the two main fragments are never connected. There are more than two fragments of the bone, which can turn into a great number of fragments if the force applied over the bone is particularly high.

Chapter Seven

Most Common Types of Fractures

In this chapter we'll take the most important fractures according to their frequency and relevance. We'll look into them individually, studying symptoms, as well as providing valuable information about treatment and recovery.

Open Fracture

This is a severe fracture because the bone breaks and pierces through the skin leading to excessive bleeding. The skin protects the inner contents of the body from exposure to all kinds of bacteria but the open fracture opens the skin, which can lead to infections in the exposed area. During open fractures, the surgeon must clean the area of the breach to avoid a bone infection. Open fractures always need surgery because there is a need to stop the bleeding and prevent contamination, which could lead to infections. Open breaches are usually severe, and there are specific steps that should be followed in such situations.

Steps to follow in the event of an open fracture

• Seek help as soon as the incidence occurs

It's best to call out for assistance whenever an incident involving a fracture occurs. There's usually a lot of blood at the scene, and the image of the protruding bone may be extremely overwhelming. The site is terrifying for many people, especially children, which may cause panic. The available people should offer the best care that they can provide, given the circumstances. However, the fracture should only be manipulated by someone trained to deal with these injuries, or else the situation can get worse.

• Call an ambulance

The patient must be taken to a hospital, straight to the emergency care unit. The patient won't be safe until someone calls for an ambulance. The ambulance will be accompanied by medical officers who will be capable of treating the wound, so if there's nobody able to give proper care to the injured patient, it's best to wait for the professional paramedics to take over the situation. Here are some vital steps to follow when on the call with the helpline:

- Provide Information on the incident.

- Keep the phone with you to ensure that there is consistent communication with the helpline.

- Listen to the precise information that is provided to be able to follow their instructions.

- It's essential to provide clear information on the location and direction of the incident.

- Once the medical team arrives, it's best to provide all the necessary information, such as how the injury happened and how long the patient has been bleeding.

- The patient's personal information should be provided to the medical team on arrival, such as the name, age, underlying diseases and allergies.

- There will be an inquiry on the actions that you have taken in managing the situation. This gives valuable information to the paramedics about the situation of the patient and the treatment he's received.

- In a situation where the incident occurred in a school, the medical report may indicate the recommended hospital that the child ought to be taken in cases of medical emergencies. The reason is that the parents may have paid health insurance in the hospital that they recommend, or maybe they work there or have a family member that works there.

- The legal guardian of the child must be informed of the incident that occurred. The parent of the child could be of critical help in cases of open fractures, the reason being that the child may need a blood transplant due to the blood loss associated with the injury. The school administration should be informed of the incident so that they can contact the parents. A record should be taken of the incident to give the parents all the necessary information.

- The decision-making process must be quick and efficient. An open fracture is a medical emergency that causes the need for one to make the best decision for the injured. The decision made has to be made quickly and efficiently.

• Administer the best first aid possible

There's usually time before the ambulance arrives, and this time should be used to provide the best care possible. As long as there's someone available that knows how to treat a fracture, this person should be in charge of providing first aid. Thankfully, if you're around, you'll know exactly what to do once you finish this book, so you'll be able to help this patient. If there's nobody else around, it's better to leave the patient alone because fractures can easily get worse.

Compression Fracture

A compression fractures have been described in the fourth chapter of this book. This kind of fracture mostly occurs in the vertebra, which is in the spine. The spine holds the body's weight against gravity, thus allowing movement and protection of the nervous system surrounded by it (the spinal cord).

Compression fractures lead to a collapse of the vertebra, which decreases their length. This collapse of the vertebra, in some cases, can suppress the supply of blood and oxygen to the spine due to the bone pieces pushing up on the spine.

There are several causes of compression fractures. One of them is osteoporosis, which causes weak bones. Some injuries occur on the vertebra due to sports, car accidents, falls, and spinal tumors.

Particular symptoms of a compression fracture in the vertebra

Symptoms that arise as a result of a compression fracture can include:

- There's a back pain that increases gradually, which gets worse when standing and decreases when lying down. If the breach happens immediately, there may be sharp, unbearable pain.

- The patient will be shorter.

- The patient's unable to do spinal movements such as bending or turning.

- The patient can't face forward in an upright manner, and he's are always in a stooped position.

- The patient may also experience a tingling sensation or numbness along the spine.

- The muscles get weak.

- The patient may experience trouble walking.

- Nerve damage could lead to problems in controlling the bladder and bowel movements.

The healthcare provider will need to perform specific tests to establish the state of the bone. These tests include X-rays, CT scans, and MRI.

Complications of a compression fracture in the vertebra

Several complications could arise from a compression fracture, such as:

- There is a possibility that the fracture may not heal well after treatment. This issue could lead to more injuries to the vertebra.

- This kind of fracture usually affects movement, which could result in blood clot formation.

- Another complication that could arise is referred to as kyphosis. This complication is an abnormality that appears on the back in the shape of a hump, which causes pain. Another consequence of these humps is that the chest organs such as the lungs and heart may develop complications.

- The nerve endings in the spine may not be recovered, leading to nerve issues along the spine.

- There may be chronic pain.

General treatment of a compression fracture

There are various ways of treating a compression fracture in the vertebra, including:

- Painkillers to reduce the pain.

- Observed physical activity to ensure that the bones heal, and there is no formation of a blood clot due to lack of movement.

- A back brace to reshape the vertebra.

- Physiotherapy to exercise the bones and make them recover their strength and mobility. This also develops the muscles that surround the bone.

- During recovery, the patient will be advised to consume foods rich in vitamin D and Calcium to strengthen the bones and promote healing.

Specialized treatment of compression fractures in the vertebra

There are situations where treatment does not work thus resulting in a need for more specialized methods of treatment.

• Vertebroplasty

The surgeon examines the radiography, which they will use for the procedure. During surgery, the surgeon will insert a needle in the fractured vertebra, which shall release a kind of cement that will support the broken area. This will lead to stability along that area and promote healing. The procedure has been reported to decrease the pain caused by compression fractures.

• Kyphoplasty

This procedure is very similar to vertebroplasty. The similarity is in the insertion of the cement in the area of the fracture. The difference is that before the infusion, miniature balloons are used to expand the broken area, thus increasing the height of the spine. The additional space created by the balloons will be filled win the special cement.

Prevention of a Compression Fracture

One of the means of preventing compression fractures is by preventing the chances of having osteoporosis. Regular health check-ups on the bones establish the bone density and are a means of identifying whether there are chances of having osteoporosis. Certain lifestyle activities increase the likelihood of having compression fractures and even cancer, such as smoking and alcohol abuse. Physical exercise is vital in the development and strengthening of bones. Accidents also lead to compression fractures; therefore, it is advisable to put measures to reduce the likelihood of the fractures occurring.

Everyday life of someone living with a compression fracture

Patients recovering from a compression fracture will need analgesics to reduce the chronic pain associated with them. Most of the compression fractures take approximately three months to heal. There are differences in the severity of the compression fractures; thus, the healing process may not be the same in all patients. If the compression fractures heal with morphological disorders, these fractures will carry consequences for the patient. There are drugs that a patient would take to reduce the chances of a fracture occurring later on in life, but these medicines do not heal fractures within the body. It is advisable for anyone who has osteoporosis to ensure that the medical complications are treated, thus preventing the likelihood of compression fractures occurring. A majority of accident-related fractures have a recovery duration of 8 weeks, but others may take longer in cases where surgery is involved. One of the consequences of cancer is that it may lead to compression fractures. The type of cancer will also determine the best way of treating the patient's compression fracture.

Skull Fracture

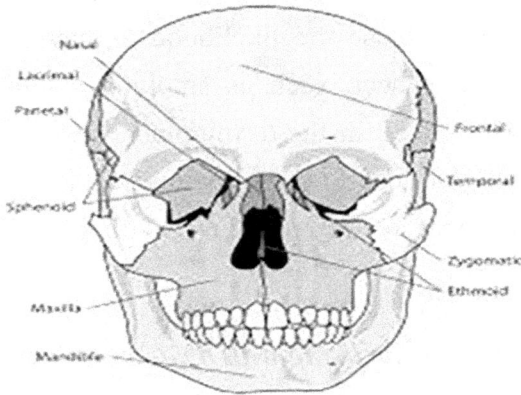

The skull is a vital part of the body because it holds and protects the brain. It takes a lot of pressure to fracture any of the bones that form the skull. In skull fractures, the biggest concern is to make sure that there's no damage to the brain. Therefore, during a possible skull fracture, a CT scan is carried out to establish that there is no damage to underlying structures, rather than a radiography.

Skull fracture symptoms are associated with blood and swelling in the injured area. These symptoms may include headaches, as well as other neurological manifestations such as numbness, hallucinations, and even seizures. Complex neurological symptoms are a sign of brain injury.

Types of skull fractures

There are different types of skull fractures, depending on the affected bone.

• Basilar skull fractures

These fractures occur at the bottom of the brain. The symptoms are usually blood coming out of the ears or nose, bruises at the back of the ear, and bruises around the eyes.

• Depressed skull fracture

The pieces of the broken bone are pushed towards the brain; surgery will always be needed, and the extension of the damage will depend on the amount of depression towards the brain tissue

• Open skull fracture

The contents of the skull are in direct contact with the external environment. Surgery must always be performed in this kind of fracture to seal the opening of the fracture. These kinds of skull fracture are particularly exposed to infections, which are a very serious complication when the affected area is considered.

Stress Fracture

A stress fracture, as described early, is also referred to as a hairline fracture. This kind of breach usually occurs after many little traumas occur on the same bone, and the bone can no longer endure the consistent stress exerted on it. The split occurs after the affected bone has been overused. These kinds of fractures tend to happen to athletes. People that have osteoporosis may also have hairline fractures, especially in the beginning stages of the condition. Whenever these microfractures have been identified, they should be treated to prevent it from turning into a complete fracture.

The absence of sufficient time for the bone to heal results in further damage from these tiny fractures resulting in a worse breach. These fractures are what leads to the permanent damage that affects athletes to the point that they can never partake in the sports activities again. However, some of the athletes that undergo severe stress fractures may recover to the extent where they can perform day to day activities, but not recover their former athletic condition.

Due to the strain of gravity, foot and leg bones are the bones that commonly suffer from hairline fractures. The bones have suffered a lot of pressure from supporting the body's weight when they performed physical activities such as running, jogging, and jumping.

The metatarsals are usually more susceptible to bone fractures. The small size of these bones makes them unable to withstand the pressure that the foot experiences from all day to day activities. These bones are mostly used when raising the foot during running or jumping. Consequently, this fracture mostly occurs amongst runners due to the repetitive pressure exerted on their feet. The bones of the body that undergo the most amount of hairline fractures are the heel, ankle, and the navicular bones.

Symptoms of hairline fractures

As explained above, the best means of healing a hairline fracture is treating the tiny fractures that occur within the body, making the early identification of stress fractures a vital part of the prevention and healing process. These are the symptoms associated with hairline fractures:

- The person will feel pain, and the degree of pain will worsen during physical activities such as weight-bearing exercises. The pain will be less when the person rests the affected segment of the body.

- The affected region may exhibit some swelling.

- There may be bruising around the site of the fracture.

Causes of stress fractures

The leading cause of stress fractures is repetitive pressure on the bone. The number of times the stress occurs, the length of its occurrence, and its degree will establish whether a stress fracture will form or not. For example, a person may have the habit of regularly going for a run, but the abrupt increment in the distance and frequency in a day or week could result in a stress fracture.

Stress fractures are also caused by a sudden change in the form of exercise that one undertakes. An example would be a person that regularly swims switching to another stressful activity such as running. The body needs to be eased slowly into performing new exercises, and this action applies to everyone despite their fitness level.

Stressful physical activities result in the replacement of old bones with new bones due to the increased breakdown, which causes hairline fractures. The act of replacing old bones with new bones is referred to as remodeling, and it can strengthen the affected bones in the long term provided they get enough rest to heal.

People at risk of suffering a stress fracture

The following are the activities and status that result in the formation of hairline fractures:

• Specific sports

Some sports particularly increase the likelihood of stress fractures due to the high rate of frequency of the pressure they apply to the body. The bone that's repetitively used in the game is the one that will be prone to the stress fracture. High-impact sports that result in athletes experiencing hairline fractures include: running marathons or track, rugby, basketball, football, tennis, dance, ballet, and gymnastics.

• Women

Women with menstrual cycle disorders are more susceptible to stress fractures. Female athletes tend to experience a strict dieting and exercise program, which affects their menstrual cycles. This kind of lifestyle for female athletes results in eating disorders. The consequence of this action is that the woman may experience the early symptomatic stages of osteoporosis, which is a fracture related disease. Over time, the athlete will have a higher likelihood of undergoing stress fractures.

• The nature of the feet

Feet come in different shapes and sizes. Some feet, depending on their shape, have an increased likelihood of developing stress fractures. Feet that have elevated arches, as well as flat feet, are more susceptible to stress fractures.

• Weak bones

Hairline fractures are a result of small fractures within the bone, so weaker bones are more prone to experiencing these fractures. Medical conditions that decrease bone density and power will lead to the person experiencing hairline fractures from performing normal daily activities such as walking and writing.

• Repetitive stress fractures

A person who has undergone a stress fracture in the past is more likely to experience a second hairline fracture. Therefore, the person should apply measures to decrease the likelihood of developing a new fracture.

• Diet

One of the reasons for hairline fractures would be the consumption of foods that do not increase the strength and density of the bones. Foods that are rich in calcium and vitamin D promote the formation of bones. There are also conditions such as eating disorders that lead to insufficient nutrient consumption, which leads to weak bones, and therefore, hairline fractures. The weather could also play an impact on the development of stress fractures. Vitamin D can be sourced from food and sunlight, which means that the cold season will lead to a low supply of vitamin D.

• Techniques used in physical activities

Inadequate athletes that exercise with a bad technique are prone to developing a stress fracture. Also, situations such as blisters can make an athlete an odd manner resulting in pressure being exerted on new areas of the foot. The sudden shift increases the likelihood of hairline fractures.

• Changing the exercise surface

In this case, the surface means the floor over which the athlete exercises. For example, jumping on grass has more cushioning that jumping on a hunk of concrete. The decreased amount of cushioning leads to more pressure being exerted on a specific region. This results in a higher chance of stress fractures on the feet and legs.

• Inadequate protective gear

The better the quality of running shoes in terms of pressure absorption, the less likely it is that such an individual could develop a hairline fracture. The pump will cushion the impact of the legs to the ground that decrease the pressure exerted, which, in turn, reduces the likelihood of stress fractures.

Diagnosis of a stress fracture

Hairline fractures can either be detected early by a routine examination, or they can be detected when the symptoms appear and the stress fracture becomes evident. In any of the cases, it can only be diagnosed by a health professional using the proper gear.

The doctor will inquire into the patient's medical history to establish whether there are underlying medical complications that have led to stress fractures such as osteoporosis. Tests will also be conducted to investigate whether there is a deficiency of bone-strengthening nutrients in the body, such as calcium. The doctor will also investigate any other causes of the fracture through interrogation, such as the patient's physical activity.

The doctor will need to perform a physical exam. He'll assess the level of pain. This test will be done by carefully applying pressure in the area suspected to have a stress fracture.

The healthcare provider will need to perform specific tests to establish the state of the bone. The other criteria that will be conducted include the following;

• Magnetic Resonance Imaging (MRI)

This is the recommended test for establishing whether a patient has a stress fracture. The MRI is preferred to the radiography because it will identify even the smallest fractures that the radiography could miss.

• **Radiography**

Stress fractures are usually very small, thus making them hard to notice with a radiography. The radiography will only reveal the stress fracture once a broken bone has produced callus in the fractured area.

• **Bone scan**

Bone scans are performed through vein infusion of radioactive material in small doses. The test is used to establish whether there is an increased blood supply to a specific region of the bones. There's usually an increased blood supply to an area where there's a broken bone. The injected substance will be drawn to the area that the body is attempting to repair. However, the method doesn't specifically isolate the type of fracture, but instead, it identifies the bone's deformity.

Complications of a stress fracture

Stress fractures are small fractures on the bone, but the repetitive pressure placed on that region could result in a complete fracture. These types of fractures tend to take much longer to heal and require much more invasive procedures. Depending on the severity of the injury, a patient may need to undergo surgery.

Recovery of stress fractures

To prevent the stress fracture turning into a full fracture, a cast is usually placed in that region.

Once the bone has healed, exercise is paramount for a quick and effective recovery because the muscles within that region need to be strengthened. The patient will be healthier active rather than sitting down for days without doing any kind of physical activity. The diet is also essential; supplying the body with the proper nutrients that strengthen bones will always contribute positively to recovery. Foods that are rich in vitamin C and Vitamin D are vital in bones recovery.

Some habits such as smoking are unhealthy during the recovery period for bone fractures, and it would be advisable to avoid. It's always advisable to quit smoking in order to improve the general health of the body.

Chapter Eight

Bone Fractures in Children

Children are very active and, therefore, susceptible to fractures. However, the examination of fractures in children is more complicated than adults because their bones have not fully developed. Children's bones have growth plates in them between the metaphysis and the epiphysis; these growth plates can be very similar to fractures, making it complicated to diagnose a fracture in them. Some physicians tend to diagnose the injury physically rather than placing reliance on a radiography in these cases in which the only available image of a possible fracture can also be confused with the growth plate.

General Information about Injuries in Children

Multiple reports have revealed that among the injuries that occur amongst people, 25% of them pertain to children. A majority of the injuries are minor medical issues, while the other injuries result in disabilities and even death. There is minimal research done on the consequences of minor injuries, but a preventive approach is recommended regarding major injuries. The major injures in children are characterized by the following:

- Injuries associated with fire leading to burns

- Consumption of poisonous substances

- Accidents that result in unconsciousness

- Brain injuries

- Possible drowning

- Fractures

Fractures in Children

The bones of the children are usually not as thick as the bones of an adult. Their compact bone tissue isn't as strong, and their bone marrow is always red bone marrow, which makes their bones easier to break. However, this also makes them more flexible, and together with the increased strength and flexibility of their periosteum, this provides a special kind of protection to children.

During our childhood, our bones are more likely to bend than break. In the case of fractured long bones, this allows two particular types of long bone fracture in children, the greenstick fracture and the buckle fracture.

Greenstick Fracture

This type of fracture gets its name by the natural shape assumed by a green stick when it's bent. It's an incomplete displaced diaphyseal fracture. One of the sides of the bone is fractured, and the other one is compressed and bent in an angle. It's not really dangerous and it can heal easily once proper treatment is applied.

Buckle Fracture

Also called a torus fracture, it's similar to a greenstick fracture but there's no actual rupture trace. The patient's bone is still bent in an angle, the affected side is compressed, but in this case, the other side isn't fractured. Just like the greenstick fracture, it's not a dangerous fracture and it can heal easily without complications. It's even safer than the greenstick fracture because there're no sharp edges to damage the surrounding structures.

The Challenge of Children

Children are, as a general rule, difficult and uncooperative patients. Their restlessness is even greater when they're in pain, so treating a child with a possible fracture becomes a true challenge. There's no great difference between the treatment of children and the treatment of adults, so the steps described in chapter eleven should still be followed. However, the immobilization, the most important step in the treatment of any possible fractures, is extremely difficult in children. For this reason, asking for external help to keep the child still and calm is, with very few exceptions, the only way to effectively treat a fractured child.

The children's parents should also be instructed to take special care of the patient during the time of recovery. Taking proper care of the cast, respecting the time of rest, and eating healthy are all activities that the child won't be able to do without help and supervision.

Chapter Nine

Vital Signs

One of the steps needed in the assessment of any polytraumatized patient is taking the vital signs, and fractured patients aren't the exception. In this chapter we'll study the right way to take the patient's pulse rate and respiratory rate.

Every clinician must run an initial assessment before treating any injured patients. This assessment must be done as quickly as possible; it has a predesigned order to follow, and it must be done correctly. Whenever dealing with a patient in a prehospital setting, paramedics do three main things. They run the assessment, they stabilize the patient, and they communicate with the health center to coordinate the hospital treatment.

Taking the vital signs is the first step of the initial assessment. Vital signs are indicators that show us the most basic body functions; this is the fastest way to assess the condition of a traumatized patient. In the case of fractured patients, the vital signs will be the only ones to tell us when the patient is in bad condition, or even in a life-threatening situation. The vital signs that we'll assess during the approach to a fractured patient are the pulse rate and respiratory rate. These provide information that will be valuable for the hospital staff. Taking these measurements shouldn't take more than sixty seconds. Fast measurements save lives and improve the patient's chance of recovery.

Respiratory Rate

This is the measure of the breaths per minute. Patients can exhibit an increased respiratory rate when they're under physical or mental stress. When the different systems of the body are shutting down, the respiratory rate can go the other way and will be under normal rates. This is indicative of a critical condition, and it's a sign of alarm. The normal respiratory rate is e between 12 and 20 breaths per minute. Lower than that is considered bradypnea, and higher than that is called tachypnea. Tachypnea over 29 breaths per minutes and bradypnea lower than ten breaths per minute should be considered a severe sign of alarm and the patient must be transferred immediately to an advanced trauma facility.

Measuring the respiratory rate

The patient can't be aware of what's going on during the measurement of the respiratory rate, or else, he may distort the reading. Breathing is observed through the movements of the expansion of the chest, abdomen, and the movements of the shoulders. If a patient's breathing is too shallow to see it, you can place your hand over the abdomen to feel its movements. You can also place your head on the patient's chest to listen to the breathing.

Counting breaths is done using a chronometer. The most reliable way to assess the respiratory rate is to count the number of breaths for one minute. However, this is too slow for an emergency. Instead, it's ideal to can count the number of breaths for thirty seconds and double that number to get the respiratory rate. You could even count them for twenty seconds and multiply that by three. You should only waste sixty seconds measuring the respiratory rate if the respirations are irregular. If the patient's breathing accelerates and decelerates constantly, you can't predict the respiratory rate with a thirty seconds measure.

Pulse Rate

Pulse rate is a vital sign that measures heartbeats. It provides valuable information regarding the patient's condition. The pulse rate can be defined as the number of times that blood is pumped through the arteries per minute. It's a reliable way to measure the patient's heart beats per minute, which is called a heart rate. The normal heart rate should be between sixty and ninety heartbeats per minute. Lower than that is called bradycardia, and higher than that is called tachycardia. An accelerated heart rate, even tachycardia, will probably be assessed in a patient under physical or mental distress. You shouldn't worry unless it reaches extremely high values. Bradycardia is the really worrying condition in any traumatized patients. Bradycardia means that the patient's heart isn't working correctly, which is a sign of alarm that shows us a poor general condition.

Measuring the pulse

The oximeter is a particular device that'll give you an automatic reading of the pulse rate, making this task much easier.

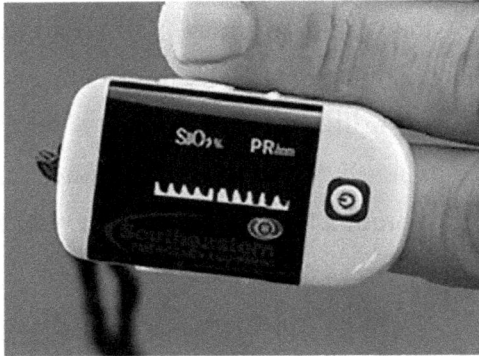

These devices are used to measure oxygen saturation in the blood. This is useful for patients with severe respiratory conditions such as pneumonia. However, oxygen saturation is not what we're looking for when we use an oximeter in a fractured patient. We want to know the pulse rate, which is also indicated by the device. You should always include one of these when you're building your first aid kit. It'll facilitate the initial assessment of the patient.

If you don't have an oximeter or any other devices able to give you a reading of the patient's blood pulse, you must learn how to measure the pulse rate yourself. It's simple enough once you understand human anatomy and the techniques behind it.

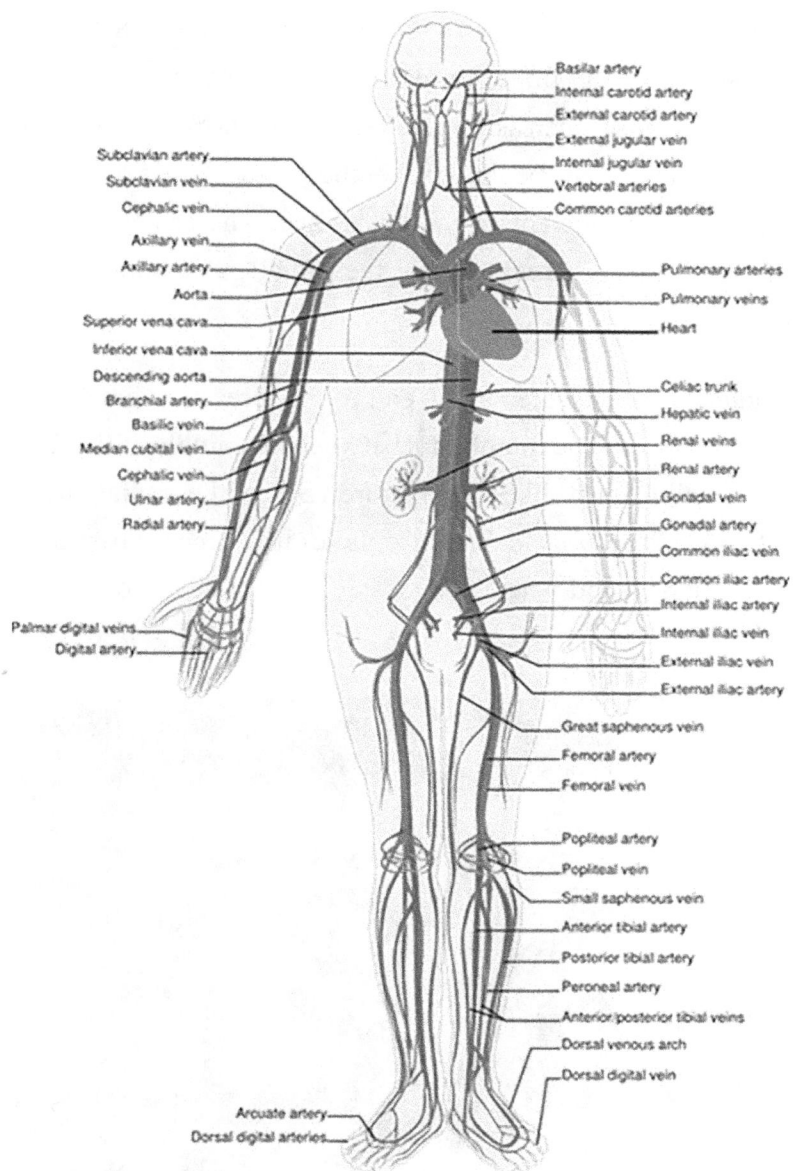

Basilar artery
Internal carotid artery
External carotid artery
External jugular vein
Internal jugular vein
Vertebral arteries
Common carotid arteries

Subclavian artery
Subclavian vein
Cephalic vein
Axillary vein
Axillary artery
Aorta
Superior vena cava
Inferior vena cava
Descending aorta
Branchial artery
Basilic vein
Median cubital vein
Cephalic vein
Ulnar artery
Radial artery

Pulmonary arteries
Pulmonary veins
Heart

Celiac trunk
Hepatic vein
Renal veins
Renal artery
Gonadal vein
Gonadal artery
Common iliac vein
Common iliac artery
Internal iliac artery
Internal iliac vein
External iliac vein
External iliac artery

Palmar digital veins
Digital artery

Great saphenous vein
Femoral artery
Femoral vein

Popliteal artery
Popliteal vein
Small saphenous vein
Anterior tibial artery
Postorior tibial artery
Peroneal artery
Anterior/posterior tibial veins
Dorsal venous arch
Dorsal digital vein

Arcuate artery
Dorsal digital arteries

The right technique to measure pulse is by using your ring, middle and index fingers. You can't use your thumb because you could confuse its pulse rate with the patient's pulse rate, gathering a wrong

223

reading. You must place these three fingers over the artery you're assessing. The ring finger is used to press over the artery and suppress the pulse, then you must release the pressure to allow the blood flow. This helps beginners feel the pulse, but it's not needed if you're already proficient in this technique. The easiest arteries to locate for pulse measurement are the radial pulse and the carotid pulse.

The radial pulse is located at the end of the forearm, right below the hand, to the side of the thumb. It's between the middle of the forearm and the radius, just like the picture. Since the radial artery is superficial, it's easy to feel a pulse there. It'll become easy for you once you understand where it's located, so this takes some practice to master.

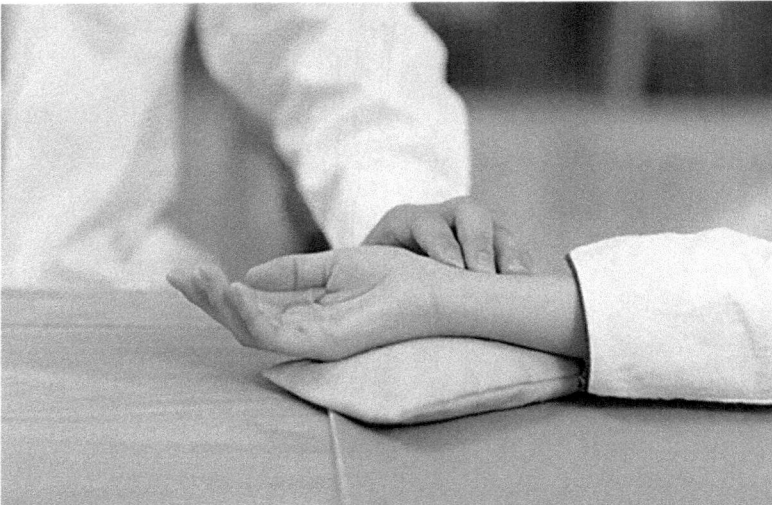

In fractured patients, the most important pulses are the ones in the limbs, to assess whether there's a compromise of the blood flow or not. So, you'll need to learn how to measure a radial pulse and a tibial pulse. Following the same technique as the radial pulse, the tibial pulse is located in the inner side of the ankle, between the achilles tendon and the posterior border of the medial malleolus (that is, the round protuberance of the tibia that's right about the feet).

Once you find the patient's pulse, count the pulsations during a lapse of sixty seconds to get the pulse rate. Similarly to the respiratory rate, this is the most reliable way to measure a pulse rate, but it's not time efficient. Since you must measure the pulse as quickly as possible, you should count the pulsations for fifteen seconds and multiply that number by four to get the desired measurement. However, if the patient's pulse is irregular and you notice it's accelerating and decelerating constantly, you the only way to measure the pulse is by counting the pulsations for sixty seconds. As a matter of fact, if the pulse is irregular, this will also affect any electronic devices designed to measure the pulse rate. In this case, you'll see the numbers go up and down constantly as the pulse rate accelerates and decelerates, so you'll need to measure the pulse manually. If the patient has a limb without a pulse, this is a critical sign that indicates the patient needs to get treatment in a trauma center immediately.

Pulses should be symmetrical. This means many things for a proficient clinician, but for an apprentice who needs to get as much information as he's able to assert, this means that the patient's pulse should be perceived as equally strong in both limbs. If the pulse of one arm is weaker than the other, that means that blood flow may have been compromised, and it's a sign for alarm. This is the reason why you should always measure both pulses in patients with a suspected limb fracture.

You should get a reading in about twenty seconds if everything's done correctly, but this can only be accomplished through practice. The best way to practice pulse measurement is by taking your own pulse.

If you're in a life-threatening or emergency medical situation, seek medical assistance immediately.

Chapter Ten

Immobilizations

Immobilizations are the cornerstone of the treatment of fractures. The only way to avoid further damage is to effectively immobilize the affected area. Patients can't be moved, much less transferred to a hospital, until they're properly immobilized. This is where most people fail at helping traumatized patients when they don't know how to treat a fracture, making the situation much worse than it should be. Paramedics who arrive at the scene will take care of immobilizing the patient before taking him to a hospital, so if you're unable to immobilize the fracture and manage the patient without moving it, it's best to leave it to the professionals. Now, since you're preparing yourself to treat a fracture, the only way to accomplish this is to study thoroughly the different immobilizations.

Types of Bandages Used in Immobilizations

These are the types of bandages you'll be using to treat fractures, so it's important to begin by learning about them.

Gauze Bandages

These are the most common and most used bandages, but not for the treatment of fractures. They're made of a woven fabric, and they're sterilized and packaged to be used. These are the bandages used to put pressure on the bleeding wounds, but also to clean and disinfect wounds. The only situation in which we should use these bandages to treat a fracture is when we place them over an open wound to cover and protect it. And even in these cases, they can't be used to apply pressure over the open wound. Since you can't move fractured bones or else you may increase the injury, you also can't apply pressure over an open fracture.

Compression Bandages

These are the bandages used to make immobilizations and improvised tourniquets. They're stronger than gauzes, but they can't absorb fluids as well as them, so they're not used to cover open fractures. Nonetheless, they're still extremely useful since they're the type of bandages you'll be using for immobilizations when you don't have specialized immobilizers.

Triangular Bandages

These are the type of bandages you'll use immobilizations in the shoulders, arms, and forearms. In case you don't have triangular bandages, you can still use compression bandages for this; however, it's still better to have triangular bandages available since they offer a wider range of applications. They're strong bandages shaped like a right-angled triangle; the tip of this triangle is called the apex of the bandage.

Tube Bandages

These are elastic bandages shaped like a tube. They're fabricated like this so we can squeeze them around limbs, allowing us to immobilize a limb by holding a strong object against the patient's affected extremity.

Tourniquets

Note: Only used if the person is at risk of bleeding to death before help arrives.

Tourniquets have a particular use in the treatment of a fractured patient. They shall only be used to stop uncontrollable bleedings in the limbs that compromise the patient's life. They're strong bandages designed to be tied around a limb and completely stop blood flow towards it. They can't be placed too long or else the limb's tissue may be damaged, but they're the only way to treat important bleedings from the limbs in fractured patients. *It's impossible to stop bleeding from the neck or torso with a tourniquet.*

Tourniquets must be placed at least two inches above the wounds. In the case of fractures, the clinician must consider placing the tourniquet even higher to avoid moving the fractured bone. Tourniquets also can't be placed over joints, so they can't go over the elbows or the knees. However, as long as the fracture's located in a distant segment of the body, it's always better to place the tourniquet in the proximal segment, thus avoiding further damage to the fracture. So, if the patient's suffering from a fracture in the forearm, it's better to place the tourniquet on the arm.

You should have at least one commercial tourniquet available in your first aid kit. These work better and are highly advisable for emergencies. Some tourniquets have inflation pumps and use them to stop the bleeding, others are designed as a belt with a strap to minimize the required force to use them. However, you'll have to use an improvised tourniquet if you don't have a commercial tourniquet at hand. Compression bandages, belts, cloth, even towels can be used as a tourniquet if nothing else is available at the moment. Start by placing the cloth material around the limb, tie it with a simple square knot, and squeeze it hard. If you can't tie the tourniquet in a way that it stops relying on your strength to remain in place, you can use a stick to help you with the tourniquet. This stick can be improvised with anything as long as it's resistant and has the right size. Once you find a stick, you must place it over the tourniquet's square knot and tie a second knot around it. Then you start spinning the stick in a clockwise direction in order to squeeze the tourniquet hard enough around the limb.

It's important to point out that tourniquets will be extremely painful and uncomfortable. A conscious patient could even beg for its removal if they're applied correctly. This is exactly the way a tourniquet must be applied, so you can't loosen the tourniquet because of the complaints of the patient.

Rules for Immobilizations

There are three main rules to apply any immobilization technique correctly.

Look for stability

The immobilization must be done with something strong to keep the affected bone in a stable position. This is where splints and cervical collars come into play. There are many commercial splints used for specific segments of the body, and it's advisable to have them all to create a safer and easier immobilization. Most of these commercial splints have their own belts and straps to be held against the fractured bone. Other splints need another kind of support to be tied around the affected limb, such as a compression bandage or a tube bandage. If you don't have a commercial splint, you may use anything suitable as an improvised splint. You can use planks, sticks, shoes, even cardboard if it's resistant enough.

The only rule for improvised splints is that they're resistant and they can be adapted to the shape of the body's segment, and tied as tightly as possible with a compression bandage (or anything else available). You can use the patient's body if you don't have anything else at hand to be used as a splint. You must attach two adjacent body segments such as legs, for example, to you make the immobilization by attaching the fractured leg to the healthy leg. You can also use the patient's torso to immobilize his arms; a triangular bandage is the best fit for these cases. There are no anatomical structures adjacent to the neck, so the patient's neck will always need any sort of object as a splint. Finding a splint to immobilize the neck is, however, an easy task. If you don't have a neck collar available, a pair of hats tied around the neck are good enough. If there are no hats available, you can even use a pair of shoes.

Secure the joints

This rule applies to limb fractures, and it's to always immobilize the proximal and the distal joint to the fracture. For example, if you want to avoid the movements in the arm, you must immobilize the shoulder and the elbow. If you must immobilize the forearm, you must immobilize the elbow and the wrist. Keep in mind that all you need to do is stabilize the limb for transportation; definitive treatment will be provided at the hospital.

Not too tight

Immobilizations must be tight enough to avoid any movements, but they can't be so tight that they change the direction of the bones, or compromise circulation or airflow. If the immobilized limb is turning pale or blue, this means that circulation is compromised, and the immobilization must be loosened. For cervical spine immobilizations, squeezing too tight will also affect the spine's position, and if the patient's face is turning pale or blue, or he's having trouble breathing, that probably means you're either compromising circulation or airflow to the head; once again, the immobilization must be loosened.

Immobilizations According to the Segment of the Body

The immobilizations must adapt to the different shapes and circumstances of the. Immobilizing an arm and a leg isn't the same thing, so the techniques to apply these immobilizations must be different.

Cervical Spine Immobilization

This is the most important immobilization because of the dangers related to cervical spine injury. Almost any traumatized patient will have a neck immobilization before he's transported to a health center. Cervical collars are the best way to make sure the patient's cervical spine is safe. They're easy to use and reliable and easy to use, so it's highly suggested to have one in the first aid kit. If you don't have a cervical collar, or any other commercial neck immobilizers, use hats, shoes, pillows, cardboard, or anything else that may adjust to the shape of the neck without forcing it to rotate to either side or tilt forward.

The process of placing a neck immobilization is very delicate, and it requires more than one person to do it. One person must lift the head and shoulders of the patient at the same time, slowly and making sure not to tilt, flex, or rotate the neck. The other person must place the immobilizer around the neck while it's lifted from the ground. Once this is in place, the patient must be placed down on the ground before securing the immobilizer in its place.

Arm Immobilizers

Arm fractures are extremely common, especially radius and ulna fractures. There are two main resources used for arm immobilization; these are splints and slings.

Splints are attached to the injured segment of the arm and they prevent it from moving. They should also try to immobilize the proximal and distal joints of the affected segment as good as possible. Commercial splints are great for support, but if none are available, any other hard materials can be used. The arm should always be immobilized with the elbow bent in a ninety degrees angle (for upper arm injuries) or tighter angle (for lower arm injuries), however, fractured arms should always be immobilized in their current position, always avoiding to move the proximal and distal joints.

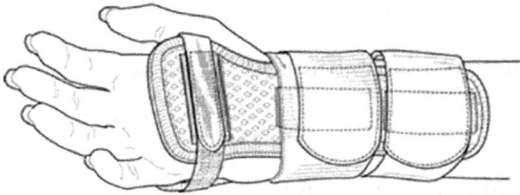

After a splint is placed, the next step is to use a sling. Slings are useful for any fractures in the arm, no matter the location. They immobilize the arms, bring stability, and even help with the bleeding if there's any. There are three types of slings you should learn and practice, so you can use them whenever they're fit. The first two need a triangular bandage or any sheet of clothing that can be bent into a triangular shape. The third one is used when there's no triangular bandage available.

The most common type of sling is the arm sling. The main focus is to immobilize the upper arm, so they're great for shoulder, humerus, clavicle, and even rib immobilization. The process of placing an arm sling starts by placing the triangular bandage under the arm, with the apex of the bandage pointing at the elbow, the longer side facing towards the feet, and the shorter side pointing at the healthy shoulder.

Once the bandage is in this position, the top side is taken behind the neck and then towards the damaged shoulder. Then, the longer side is taken up, over the patient's forearm, and towards the damaged shoulder where it meets the tip of the bandage's shorter side. Both tips are tied together and then the corners of the knot are tucked down below the bandage. The arm and forearm should be already in the right position by this point, with the forearm placed horizontally with a slight elevation towards the hand. Then, the sling is finished by extending the bandage towards the little finger, providing support from the elbow to the fingertips. Then, the apex of the bandage is tied behind the elbow to improve stability.

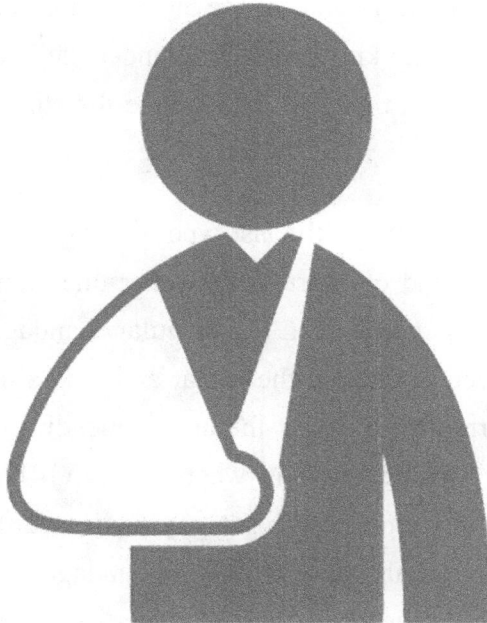

The second kind of sling is the elevated arm sling. This sling is a great fit for lower arm injuries, so it's used in forearm, wrist, and hand injuries. Since it elevates the forearm towards the healthy shoulder, it's great at reducing forearm and hand bleeding. However, if there's suspicion of a fractured bone, it's best not to bend the elbow in such an acute angle unless the arm is already positioned that way. The process of applying this type of sling begins by placing the injured forearm diagonally over the chest, with the fingertips towards the healthy shoulder. Then the triangular bandage is placed over the arm with the apex over the elbow and one of the ends over the healthy shoulder. The bandage's lower end is then tucked under the forearm and the elbow. The bandage's free end is taken behind the patient's back and directed diagonally towards the healthy elbow, where it meets the other end. Both ends of the bandage are tied together, and then the corners of the knot are tucked under the bandage. Finally, the bandage's apex is tied shut to improve the stability behind the elbow.

The collar-and-cuff sling is the last type of sling. It doesn't provide as much stability and comfort as the other ones, but it's the only available sling if there aren't triangular bandages. If you've successfully placed a splint, the collar-and-cuff sling is easier to adapt to the current position of the arm, depending on the patient. This is ideal for fractured patients where the arm is far from a flexed position. It uses a compression bandage or any sort of cloth that can be folded until it resembles a compression bandage. The center of the compression bandage is placed behind the patient's neck and healthy shoulder, and both ends of the bandage must be pointing down towards the arm. Place the arm in the desired position (the same position in which you found it, if you suspect it to be fractured. Finish the sling by taking both tips around the wrist and tying a knot below it.

It's important to assess the circulation in order to make sure it's not compromised by the sling or the splint, once they're placed. The way to assess circulation is by squeezing one of the fingertips of the affected arm. The fingertip should turn pale under the pressure because it's no longer receiving blood. If the fingertip recovers its color in under three seconds after the pressure's released, then there's no compromise in the circulation of the arm; if it doesn't, the immobilization should be assessed and done again. Of course, if there's massive blood loss or a tourniquet placed on the arm, circulation assessment is impossible.

Leg Immobilization

Immobilizing a leg is less complicated than immobilizing an arm in an emergency. The ideal position of an immobilized leg is with the knee joint slightly flexed. The patient's leg can't be completely straight during immobilization, but it can't be too flexed either. Sometimes it helps to place a small roll of bandage under the knee to procure this slight flexion of the leg. When it comes to the ankle, the angle between the leg and the foot should be of ninety degrees. Most commercial leg splints already come prepared to keep the leg and foot in the right position, but if there's no commercial splint available, improvising a splint to the back of the leg should be enough to get the desired effect. These immobilizations also use compression bandages to keep the splint attached to the leg. Remember that you can use the healthy leg as a splint for the injured leg. The paramedic should also check the circulation of the leg to be sure it's not compromised the same way the circulation of the arm is assessed. Fractured legs should follow the general rule of avoiding to move the proximal and distal joints of the fracture.

Thoracic and Lumbar Spine Immobilization

There's no splint big enough to immobilize the lumbar or thoracic spines. Fractures in these locations could also harm the spinal cord, so any suspected injuries must be taken seriously.

Professional paramedics have a stretcher to immobilize thoracic and lumbar spine, this is the reason why it's always better to wait for the paramedics as long as there's hope that they'll arrive at the scene. The stretcher will be lowered until it's right next to the patient's body, then they work in groups to lift the patient and place him over the stretcher, making sure to avoid any rotations and flexions of the spine. Once the patient is in the stretcher, he's secured with straps to keep his torso from rotating, flexing and extending. That's the last step of the immobilization before getting the patient into the ambulance and transporting him to a health center; the cervical spine must already be immobilized before this.

You probably won't have a stretcher at hand if you're on your own. The best option to give the patient a safe transport to the health center is to wait for the paramedics; however, if you know there won't be paramedics and you must take charge of the transportation yourself, you should make your best effort to avoid lumbar and thoracic spine movements. When you get ready to lift the patient to the vehicle, ask for help. If you're lifting the head and shoulders, one or two more helpers lifting the torso, and one last person lifting the legs by the ankles, you should be able to carefully move the patient while avoiding spine movements. If the amount of help available is limited or non-existent, you must make your best effort with what you have available. Remember that this is the last step of immobilization, so cervical spine should already be in place.

If you're in a life-threatening or emergency medical situation, seek medical assistance immediately.

Chapter Eleven

Broken Bones and Emergencies

The skeletal system has 204 different bones, and in some cases, it may be difficult to examine with the naked eye whether one of these is fractured or not. An example would be a person who is in excruciating pain in the neck, back or head. Such fractures would not be as easily visible as those that take place on the limbs. Fractures can be identified by the clinic exhibited by the patient and whenever the clinician suspects a fracture, the patient must be treated as a fractured patient.

General Rules for the Treatment of a Fracture

No matter the type and location of the fracture, there are simple steps that must always be followed for someone who aims to provide treatment to a fractured patient.

Call an ambulance

This is the first thing anyone should do in front of an injured person in need of help. You can't proceed to treat the patient until you're certain that someone around you is actively trying to contact an ambulance. An ambulance from the nearest hospital will arrive quickly to attend to the person with a fracture or any other medical emergencies.

These are the essential points to follow when you're calling an ambulance:

- Inform the helpline of the incident that occurred.

- Make sure that you don't abandon the phone amid all the commotion.

- Carefully listen to the instructions provided by the person in the helpline.

- Inform the person of your exact location and the means of getting there if inquired.

- Where necessary, you can assign someone to meet the medical team once they arrive to guide them to the patient's exact location.

- Upon the arrival of the medical team, be sure to give them all the necessary information.

- Inform the medical team of the name, age, and sex of the patient, as well as whether the patient has any allergies, medical conditions, the treatment provided, and the vital signs assessed.

- In the case of an injured patient in an institution, such as a school, these institutions usually have medical records of their students; hence, the school should supply this information to the medical team.

- The person on the phone will need a description of the wounded area and possible injury, to provide this to the medical. They'll also need this information upon arrival at the scene.

- There will be an inquiry on the actions that you have taken in managing the situation to make ensure that you're doing the right thing or whether you should do something else to aid the patient.

Call the medical personnel of the institution, if possible

If the patient's located in an institution, or close to an institution such as a school, usually there's medical staff that should be contacted and brought for help.

Seek assistance

Treating a fractured patient requires more than one pair of hands, so it's important to ask for assistance between those around the patient that are able to help. The person with the knowledge must always take charge of the situation, providing clear instructions on how to help treat the patient. This takes confidence, so it's important to have a good grasp of what's to be done in order to have a clear head when the moment arrives. Easy tasks such as bringing medical supplies, contacting the ambulance, bringing out the supplies and handing them over, and holding the patient in place can be trusted to those around the acting paramedic.

Call the legal guardian when a child is involved

The legal guardians must be informed of the incident, as well as the hospital where they'll that they will find their child. In a situation where the parents do not pick up the phone, the child must still be rushed to the hospital and the legal guardians informed later. The school's staff should be informed of the incident so they can keep trying to contact the legal guardians. This isn't just because of empathy for the legal guardian. Legal guardians can take care of any financial needs, as well as provide blood transfusions if the patient needs them.

Immobilizations

Until the suspected fractures are properly immobilized, the patient can't be moved at all. The only acceptable exception for this rule is when the patient's located in a dangerous area. In this case, the patient has to be moved to a safe place for both the patient and the paramedic.

The rationale behind this is that the movement of the person might worsen the possible fracture. An incomplete fracture can turn into a complete fracture, a non-displaced fracture can turn into a displaced fracture, the edges of the fracture can harm the surrounding organs, and the fracture can deteriorate in many other ways if movement or pressure if applied before immobilizing the patient.

Make decisions in the best interest of the patient

As stressful as these situations may be, it's important to maintain a clear head and make the right decisions for the patient. If the conditions aren't suitable, for example, a patient located in a place where he's in imminent danger, then the priority becomes moving the patient from there, even before applying the immobilization. The process of decision-making must be fast and efficient in order to help the patient in the best way possible.

Administer First Aid When Necessary

There are a few things that you can do while y0u wait for the ambulance to arrive. These steps will be described in the following segment of this chapter, but you can start with the initial assessment and immobilization. It's important to point out that the patient's not to be transported to the hospital is there's professional help on the way that's able to do that.

Treating a Broken *Bone* by Yourself

Sometimes you won't have professional help anywhere near you, and the only one able to treat the fractured patient, while the professional help is on the way, will be you. Sometimes professional help will be even impossible, depending on the location of the accident and the general situation around you, so you'll be the one responsible for preparing the patient for transportation and taking him to a hospital. An example of this situation would be an accident in the wilderness, such as a camping accident. This is exactly the situation that this book is preparing you for, and these are the general steps that you should follow in these cases.

Approaching the patient

The means of approaching the patient can be divided into 3 ways, which are the scene survey, the primary survey, and the secondary survey.

The scene survey looks into the identification of other possible threats. If the patient's located in a dangerous place, then the first step is to move the patient to a safe place, before anything else.

The primary survey would be looking around to identify anyone that may assist you with the patient. One of those around you should keep actively trying to contact professional help, even if it's impossible to receive.

Finally, the secondary survey looks into the physical examination of the patient, identifying the wounds, measuring the vital signs, and assessing the condition of the patient. Then, the wounds are treated and patient's immobilized. The secondary survey will be expanded in the following segment of this chapter.

Treating the wounds

Once the wounds have been identified, they must be rated by the level of danger they represent to the patient's condition, and dealt with in order.

Large bleedings must be assessed first. If there are open fractures causing an important bleeding, gauze bandages must be used to cover the open fracture. It's important to point out that, even if there are open fractures bleeding, you can't apply pressure over the wound.

Applying pressure over a fractured bone can only worsen the situation, so the only thing you can do is cover the wound with gauze bandages to create a seal.

If there are no large bleedings, or large bleedings have already been dealt with, the next step is to apply the immobilizations. It may seem counterintuitive, but immobilizing the neck always comes before immobilizing the segments of the body that seem affected by a fracture. This is because neck injuries can be hard to diagnose, they're extremely dangerous, and any movements during the immobilization of the other segments of the body may change the neck's position. Once the neck has been immobilized, the affected segments of the body are immobilized. Immobilizations have been described in the previous chapter of this book.

This is as far as the treatment of any fracture goes in a prehospital setting. The clinician's ends when the fractured segment of the body is adequately immobilized, thus preventing further damage and deterioration of the fracture. Other injuries such as muscle strains and joint dislocations can be very similar to fractures, and they're treated the same way, so if the injury seems to be a fracture, but the patient's uncertain, then clinician should still immobilize the affected segment of the body and take the patient to the nearest hospital.

Prevent shock

Once the wounds have been treated, the next step is to try to keep the patient's body temperature to avoid hypothermia and shock. The patient is covered by a space blanket, a thermal blanket, a wool blanket, or anything else available to keep the patient's temperature from dropping. This is the reason why it's advised to have space blankets in the first aid kit.

Evacuation

If there's no professional help on the way, the patient must be taken to the nearest hospital available. If all measures and treatment have been applied correctly, the patient's going to be safe.

The contents of this book must be studied thoroughly, and a medical kit should be readily according to the instructions of this book to increase the chance of the patient's survival and recovery.

If you're in a life-threatening or emergency medical situation, seek medical assistance immediately.

Chapter Twelve

Repairing a Broken Bone

The ultimate aim after a fracture is that the bone should heal well by returning to the position it once was before the injury.

Before the doctor can apply the best treatment for the patient, the doctor will need the following from the patient:

The patient's medical history to establish whether there are any pre-existing conditions such as HIV/AIDS, amongst others. The medical history will also determine the blood type of the patient to ensure that there is extra blood for the patient, especially where there is excessive bleeding or to prevent blood loss during surgery.

The patient needs to inform the doctor of any medicine or supplement that they are taking and the medicine that they may be allergic to, which includes over the counter medication.

In broken bones, there must be an imaging test done to establish the type of fracture and the precise position of the broken bone. Imaging tests include MRI scans, CT scans, and X-rays.

Where the doctor recommends surgery, the patient must not eat anything 8 hours before surgery.

It is also recommended that someone should be available to take the patient home after the procedure.

The means or repairing a broken bone will depend on the severity of the fracture, which will be established by the doctor. The place where the fractured has occurred within the body will also be important in determining the best treatment.

Severe fractures usually take much longer to heal and require much more invasive procedures such as bone grafting. Another invasive procedure is open reduction and internal fixation surgery, which is typically a surgical procedure using pins, rods, and metal screws to repair the broken bone. Less severe fractures are usually treated with a cast to align the bone and enhance healing of the broken area.

Open Reduction and Internal Fixation Surgery

This type of surgery is usually done where a cast has previously been used, but the broken bone will not heal after a cast has been used. The surgeon typically recommends this procedure before the placement of a cast, depending on the severity of the fracture.

Cases that require open reduction and internal fixation surgery are where the bone is protruding out of the skin. These kinds of broken bones are referred to as compound fractures. Broken bones on the ankles, wrists, and joints also tend to rely on this form of treatment because they are areas that could severely affect the casualty's ability to move that region.

The Negative Consequences of Bone Repair

The risks involved in bone repair surgery are not very common, but the following are a few of the complications that could arise.

A patient could end up not reacting to the anesthesia positively, thus leading to adverse side effects and the inability to be woken up from the anesthesia. This risk is a general surgical concern that could happen in any surgical procedure.

There could be excessive bleeding during the surgery, which could result in death.

There is the possibility of a blood clot occurring, which could cost the life of the patient.

An infection could arise during surgery, especially if they're the surgical equipment is not well sanitized.

Some of the complications attached to this surgery could be avoided once the doctor is made aware of the patient's medical history. The difficulties could arise in any operation, not specifically to bone repair, but that does not make them any less of a risk when one undergoes surgery.

The Means of Performing Bone Fracture Surgery

A surgeon may need a couple of hours to perform this kind of surgery. The first step would the anesthesiologist administering anesthesia to the patient. There two types of anesthesia.

This type of anesthesia places the patient in a deep sleep during the surgery.

• Local Anesthesia

This type of anesthesia makes the area where the surgery is to be performed to be numb to ensure that there is no pain, but the patient is awake during the surgery.

• General Anesthesia

This type of anesthesia places the patient in a deep sleep throughout the surgery.

The surgeon identifies the position of the incision above the fracture for the placement of a screw or plate.

An incision is made beneath a long bone, followed by the placement of a rod underneath it to give it stability and treat the fracture. This action ensures that the broken bone is appropriately positioned, and this is done using pins, rods, metal screws, or plates. These items used in securing the bone could be permanent or temporary. The surgeon will also repair the blood vessels that got injured as a result of the surgery.

Once the broken bone has been adequately secured, the incision is closed using staples or stitches. The incision wound upon closure is wrapped in sanitized dressing to reduce the chances of an infection.

Once the surgical procedure is completed, a cast may be placed on the injured area.

There would be some extreme damages to the bone, for example, if the bone were extremely shattered to which the doctor would recommend a bone transplant. This technique is referred to as bone grafting, which is a concept that we shall soon establish.

Post Bone Fracture Repair

Once the surgery is completed, the medical staff will take the patient to the recovery room to monitor their vitals, such as blood pressure, temperature, and breathing. There will be consistent check-ups while in the recovery room to ensure that the surgery did not bring about any complications such as an infection

The doctor will explain to the patient the approximate time it would take to heal the broken bone based on how the surgery went. The time that the fracture will take to heal varies due to factors such as different types of fractures and affected bones.

The hospital admission will depend on the severity of the injury and the type of surgery. The duration of the hospitalization will also depend on the rate of the patient's recovery while at the hospital.

Surgeries are typically painful afterward, but the medical staff will supply painkillers to reduce the pain. There's usually some swelling, which will be monitored as well to ensure it's not abnormal. Elevation of the fractured limb will decrease the swelling, and ice will only be used as long as there's not a cast.

Before the discharge, the doctor will instruct the patient on the means of managing their stitches and staples. This information is essential to ensure that the stitched-up wound does not open up, for example, due to excessive physical activity much sooner than prescribed. One other rule is that the area where the surgery is performed should be very hygienic to decrease any chances of an infection.

The doctor will also instruct the patient on the check-ups after discharge from the hospital; this is to ensure that the healing process is going well.

There are three stages of bone healing, and they are as follows:

• Reactive Stage

After a fracture, there usually the formation of a blood clot around the injured area. This blood clot structures itself in a way that builds a bridge to fill in the spaces that are between the two broken bones. This process aids in the combination of the bone that has been split into two.

• Repair Stage

This stage is focused on strengthening the bone once again. There are specialized cells that are found on the exterior part of the bone, which creates cartilage. This cartilage transforms into a bone referred to as a callus that pulls the bones together to make it one healthy bone once more.

• Remodeling Stage

Past the repaid stage, the patient can move around again because the bone has its strength once more. The remodeling stage is for shaping the bone to return to its previous size.

After the surgery, the patient may be able to feel the plate or screw that was installed during the surgery, especially where there is minimal muscle or soft tissue that is concealing them. Areas that would have the slightest amount of muscle or tissue covering them would be the ankle or the upper part of the hand.

Once the broken bone has healed, the doctor will recommend that installed items such as screws or plates be removed, especially where they are causing an irritation. The irritation shouldn't be a significant concern because it can be caused by external factors such as the plate rubbing against the shoe after an ankle bone repair surgery.

It is also be recommended that one undergoes physiotherapy after a bone repair surgery to strengthen the bone, thus increasing the rate of recovery. Due to the patient being dormant after the surgery, muscles around that region ought to be stretched via physical exercise. These exercises will improve the healing process and ensure that there shall be no injuries that can occur in that region that can be affiliated to the broken bone.

There are blood vessels that are linked to bones, which increase the healing process of a fracture. During the healing process, your body will form new blood vessels using the blood cells of the body to aid in healing the broken bone.

It is essential to follow the instructions given by the doctor to prevent another fracture from occurring on the same bone. It can happen in two ways. The first would be to ensure that the time when the doctor instructs the patient to begin physiotherapy on the broken bone should be followed. A patient that goes ahead and starts too soon man stand at a risk of furthering the unhealed fracture. The second means would be after the recovery of the broken bone. It would be advisable to exercise caution to prevent multiple fractures from occurring on the same bone over time.

Diet is also critical during the recovery period of a bone fracture. Certain foods have nutrients that specifically strengthen bones. Foods that are rich in calcium and Vitamin D would be recommended during the recovery period.

Some doctors would also recommend the patient to wear protective gear to decrease the chances of another fracture, such as wearing helmets, braces, or pad.

Chapter Thirteen

Additional Options for Repairing a Broken Bone

Emergency care refers to the primary means one could use to repair a broken bone, but other options are available where the primary means do not suffice.

Bone Grafting

Bone grafting is a method of bone repair that involves the transplantation of bone tissue to fix a damaged bone. Only a qualified surgeon performs this method.

Bone grafting is used in the placement of an implanted device in the position of the bone; the bone grows around the device, ensuring enhancement of bone formation. This technique is used in total knee replacement in cases of a fracture or the loss of a bone.

The transplanted bone can be sourced within the body of the injured person, a donor, or synthetic placement. The bone transplant provides a framework where new, living bone can grow around the implant to enhance bone repair.

Types of Bone Grafts

There are many types of bone grafting methods, and their applications depend on the circumstances of the case. Nonetheless, two types are very common, and they are as follows;

• Allograft

This form of bone graft uses the transplanted bone of a deceased person to the recipient in need of a bone transplant. The bone is cleaned and placed in a tissue bank for preservation until the day of surgery. This method is mostly applicable to the knee, hip, and long bone (bones in the arms or legs) reconstructive surgery.

The benefit of this method is that the injured will not have to undergo another surgery to obtain a bone within their body. A decrease in the number of operations lowers the chances of infection, which could be fatal. Another advantage of this method is that there are no living cells within the bone, thereby decreasing the possibility of the body rejecting the transplant. The absence of living bone marrow increases the chances of success because the blood type of the donor and the recipient is inconsequential.

• Autograft

Autograft bone graft is sourced from the body of the injured person, which means a bone is obtained from another part of the body. An example would be from the ribs.

The Need for Bone Grafting

The severity of the fracture case will determine the need for bone grafting i.e., the more serious the case, the more likely that bone grafting will be a treatment. Below are a few examples where bone grafting was a solution to a fracture:

- Despite emergency care being beneficial, some fractures are complicated, for example, where there are numerous fractures. These types of fractures usually don't heal very well in the beginning; therefore, a bone transplant would be necessary.

- Spinal fusion requires bone grafting for it to be done. This bone graft is because a surgeon will need an additional bone to join the two bones together, thus creating one bone where there is an area that has a disease or is injured. These conjoined bones will, therefore, be stimulated to heal by fusing.

- Bone grafting aids bones in recovering where there is a surgery that has required the implantation of devices, for example, during joint replacement.

- Bone grafting aids bone regeneration, for example, where a bone has been injured or infected. The revival can be stimulated by the use of a little bone from bone cavities or taking out a large portion size of bone depending on the need of the patient.

The Negative Consequences of Bone Grafting

There are very many risks that are attached to surgical procedures that could result in death. Therefore, it is recommended that an injured person should be adequately taken care of through emergency care to avoid surgery. Some of the risks that are attached to operations are as follows:

- Excessing bleeding during the operation.

- An infection during surgery

- There are adverse reactions to the anesthesia delivered during surgery.

- There are specific risks attached to bone drafting, and they are as follows;

- Excessive pain post-surgery. There are painkillers in place to reduce the pain, but there will still be pain afterward.

- The surgery could result in nerve damage, which could result in the inability to use that bone; for example, complications during spinal fusion could result in paralysis.

- The bone could reject the transplanted bone.

- There could be abnormal inflammation in the area where bone grafting surgery was performed.

Preparations for Bone Grafting

Bone grafting is a type of surgery, which means specific preparations must be made beforehand to perform it. The following are the preparations that must be put in place:

A medical history of the patient will be necessary to know whether the patient will be the right candidate for bone grafting surgery. A current physical exam would also need to be done to establish the health status of the patient.

The patient would also need to inform the doctor of any medicine that they are taking before the surgery.

Before surgery, one cannot consume anything because of the risk of vomiting and choking to death on the surgical table during surgery because they will be under anesthesia.

The doctor will also inform the patient of any other things that they ought to do before the surgery, which the patient must follow.

The hospital will provide a gown to the patient to wear during the surgery. There will be a tube inserted in your arm, referred to as an intravenous line. The patient will be placed on the operating table. A urinary catheter will be placed in the patient.

The Means of Performing Bone Graft Surgery

Before landing on the surgical table, there will be some appointments done to discuss with the doctor the best type of bone grafting surgery to be done and the reasons behind that. The doctor will also inform the patient about the likelihood of success and failure of the surgery.

Before surgery, an anesthesiologist will put the patient in a deep sleep by administering anesthesia. After surgery, the anesthesiologist will wake the patient.

During surgery, the area where the bone transplant will be placed will be identified, and an incision will be done right over that area. The incision will then be shaped in a manner that will fit the bone transplant. The bone transplant will be secured using the following tools:

- Wires

- Cables

- Pins

- Plates

- Screws

Upon holding the bone transplant in place, the incision made will be closed using stitches, and the wound will be sealed with bandages. A cast will be placed on that area to offer it support and ensure that the bone heals. However, a cast or a splint is not used in all cases unless there is a necessity.

Post Bone Grafting Surgery

The healing process after surgery will not be at the same rate for all bone grafting surgery. The recovery rate of the surgery will depend on many factors, such as the size of the bone transplant. Generally, most bone grafting patients recover in 2 weeks, while others may take a year or more. The surgeon will instruct that the patient should not place pressure on the area where the surgery has taken place for some time.

It is recommended that the bone graft area should have ice applied to it and elevated to ensure that the bone grafted area does not swell because if it does, it would be painful and blood clot could form. Blood clots on the skin are essential because they prevent excessive bleeding, but if they form within the veins, they could stop blood flow to organs such as the lungs or heart, which would be fatal to a patient. The main rule is that a patient who has undergone a bone transplant to the arm or leg ought to elevate those regions above their heart. Where a cast has been placed, ice should be placed on top of the cast to reduce any swelling.

Exercise is paramount for a quick and effective recovery because the muscles within that region need to be strengthened. The patient will be healthier active rather than sitting down for days without doing any kind of physical activity. The diet is also essential, supplying the body with the proper nutrients that strengthen bones will also contribute positively to recovery.

Some habits such as smoking are unhealthy during the recovery period, and it would be advisable to quite to improve the health status of the body. Liran Levin and Devorah Schwartz- Arad published an article explaining that smoke decreases the healing process and growth of bones. They illustrated that smokers that undergo bone graft surgery tend to fail far much more than non-smokers. Some surgeons do not perform bone graft surgery on smokers because of the higher failure rate.

Knee Replacement Surgery

The other name for this kind of surgery is arthroplasty or total knee replacement. The purpose of the procedure is to fix a damaged knee. The cause for the needs of this surgery could be bone-related diseases leading to arthritis. Another cause would be trauma from accidents. A lot of external pressure being exerted on the knee, which leads to post trauma-arthritis. The surgery is only necessary as a means of relieving pain or a deformity that has arisen from arthritis or knee injury. There are multiple forms of knee-related arthritis, and they include:

• Osteoarthritis Arthritis

This type of arthritis is common amongst the elderly and middle-aged people and is caused by the degeneration of the joints. This degeneration affects the joint cartilage and the nearby bones in the knees.

• Rheumatoid Arthritis

This type of arthritis leads to swelling of the synovial membrane leading to a lot of synovial fluid being retained inside the membrane. This action causes a lot of pain and makes the joint stiff affecting movement.

• Traumatic Arthritis

As earlier explained, trauma arthritis is associated with trauma injuries from accidents. They arise when significant force or impact is exerted on the knee leading to the cartilage of the bone being damaged.

The Analysis of the Knee

The knee has a joint, which is a linkage of two bones. The purpose of joints is to facilitate movement hence their mobile characteristic. The knee is composed of two long bones that are stuck together with muscles, tendons, and ligaments. Tendons are cords made of very tough connective tissues that link muscles to bones. Ligaments are elastic bands that join one bone to another. There are knee ligaments that secure the joints and ensure that the joints are stable. There are also knee ligaments that limit the mobility of the shin bone, also known as the tibia, when it comes to forward and backward movement. The 2 bones have a top layer of cartilage, which is for shock absorption to prevent knee damage.

Two forms of muscles are found in knees, and they are as follows:

• Quadriceps Muscles

They are found in front of the thighs. Their sole purpose is to align the legs.

• Hamstring Muscles

This is found behind the thighs. They are the muscles human beings use when bending or squatting using the knee.

The Composition of the Knee

• Tibia

As earlier mentioned, this is the shin bone, which is the long bone that goes down past the knee to the ankles.

• Femur

This is the thigh bone, which is a long bone that moves from the waist down to the knee.

• Patella

This is the scientific term for the kneecap.

• Cartilage

As earlier explained, cartilage is a form of tissue that is found in bones. In this case, cartilage is found at the top layer of the bone at the joint, which is the knee region. Cartilage reduces friction that arises from mobility within the joint.

• Synovial Membrane

This is a type of tissue that borders the knee joint and contains it in a joint capsule. The membrane contains a clear fluid referred to as the synovial fluid that is released to lubricate the joint.

• Tendon

This is a connective tissue that links muscles to the bones and manages the mobility of the joint.

• **Meniscus**

This is the part of the joint that absorbs shock.

The Need for the Procedure

The need for knee replacement surgery is to decrease the pain and deformity that is on the knee. As mentioned above, there are various reasons as to why one may need knee replacement surgery. Nonetheless, the most prevalent reason would be the condition referred to as Osteoarthritis.

Any damage to the cartilage and bone affects the mobility of a human being, and is an extremely painful experience. The people that suffer from any of the above-mentioned knee-related arthritis have difficulty in the movement that involves the knee. Such patients tend to have a challenge performing everyday activities such as walking, going up the stairs, jogging, running, kneeling, or even sitting. A lot of pain usually accompanies these activities. The knee tends to appear inflamed because of the instability within the joint.

Arthritis leads to the degeneration of the knee joint, or it could arise from an accident that causes severe injury to the knee. In the case of broken bones, ripped cartilage, and ligaments, the damage tends to very severe to the point that it cannot be repaired, forcing the need for knee replacement surgery.

There are usually other medications that a person who has knee-related arthritis, but in the absence of successful recovery, then knee replacement surgery becomes the solution. A few examples of these treatments are as follows.

• Physiotherapy

This is used to strengthen the bones around the knee as a means of recovery. It is usually with the aid of a physiotherapist to ensure that the exercises in place do not end up worsening the injury.

• Pain Killers

As mentioned above, knee-related arthritis is very painful, so doctors inclusive of other medication prescribe pain medication as well.

• Anti-Inflammatory Medication

This is medication to reduce the swelling caused by arthritis, which causes pain.

• Reduction in Physical Movement

A physiotherapist usually monitors physiotherapy. However, some movements are day to day which should be avoided in cases of knee-related arthritis. The reason for this to prevent the damage from worsening.

• Weight Loss

The joints of the knee are a combination of 2 long bones. These bones support a lot of the weight of the body. In cases of knee arthritis, the weight should support be decreased due to damage to the knee joints. This will reduce the amount of weight being supported, especially for people who are obese.

• Assisting Devices

It is necessary to reduce the amount of pain and pressure being exerted on the knee joints when performing daily activities. An example would be using canes for walking so that some of the weight is supported by the cane, thus reducing the weight being held by the knee joints.

• Injection of Lubrication Agents

As earlier explained, there is usually friction that occurs within the knee joints from the movement, which is absorbed within the knee to prevent pain. Damage to the knee can lead to the friction absorption limitation, thus increasing the amount of pain experienced as a result of movement. Some injections are done to lubricate the joints, thus limiting the friction and reducing the pain. These injections are referred to as visco-supplementation

Risks Involved in Knee Replacement Surgery

There are always risks that are attached to any surgical procedure, but that does not mean that there will be no success. There have been very successful knee replacement surgery procedures. Despite the success, complications can arise including fractures.

The procedure, if not done well, may lead to another fracture within the knee, which would be extremely painful to the patient.

• Consistent Pain and Constraint in Movement

The procedure will be very painful afterward, and the patient may have difficulty in doing movements that are associated with the knee.

The pain that was there as a result of the knee related injury will not be addressed using surgery, but once the joint heals then, it will decrease gradually.

There are innervated with nerves and blood vessels that are in the knee region. After a severe knee-related injury, theses nerves and blood vessels are usually damaged, which causes weakness and paralysis in that region.

This is not a conclusive list of all the complications that could arise from a knee replacement surgery procedure, but they are some of the issues that arise.

Post-Discharge

The patient must ensure that the surgical region is cleaned and dry to prevent any bacteria from arising. The surgeon will give the patient a program on how frequent the cleaning should be done. After some hospital check-ups, the doctor will remove the stitches and the staples that were used in closing up the incision during surgery.

The doctor will instruct the patient to ensure that their legs are raised, and ice is placed on the leg to ensure that the surgical area does not swell.

Complications could arise after surgery, and it is vital to inform the doctor of any changes in the body. Various symptoms could arise post-surgery and below are a few examples:

- A fever- in some cases this would be a sign that the patient is suffering from an infection

- Inflammation of the surgical area.

- Change in color of the surgical area such as redness

- Sudden bleeding

- Other fluids being released from the surgical are

- Excessive pain in the surgical area

The doctor may also recommend a diet plan for the patient to ensure a quick recovery. The patient will be having medical checkups and physiotherapy after the surgery. These activities ensure that the recovery of the patient will go smoothly. After the recovery of the patient, the doctor will then approve whether the patient is capable of certain activities or not such a driving.

The recovery period of a patient that has undergone knee replacement surgery can take a couple of months.

After surgery, it is advised that the patient avoid strenuous activities and avoid situations that could result in a fall. Some accidents could occur while in the house, which can damage the knee replacement. This creates a need to ensure that there a safety protocol installed or removed in the house for a person that has undergone knee replacement surgery. The house adjustments that should be made include:

- A chair or bench should be placed in the shower to assist the patient when showering.

- A reaching stick to allow the patient to access high areas within the house without having to stretch out the knee.

- Any loose rug that someone can trip over should be removed, and uneven floors should be fixed.

- An elevated toilet seat is recommended to decrease the bending that will be exerted on the knee because it is still in recovery.

- Areas where people move a lot, such as to the bedroom, bathroom, and kitchen, should be open and transparent. Items such as furniture and extension cords should not be present in this region to reduce the chances of tripping over them.

- Bathrooms tend to be wet, which means that that the floor should be non-slippery, and there must be non-slippery mats as well.

- Carrying the patient up the stairs in the absence of ramp. This act reduces the bending motion exerted on the knee and the likelihood of a fall occurring.

- The shoes worn should have a firm grip on the ground, and the floor should not be made out of slippery material.

- Handrails when going and down the stairs are needed for extra support.

Chapter Foruteen

Fracture Prevention

S ome people have lived their whole lives without ever breaking a bone in their body. This disparity can be attributed to luck and significant genes for some people, exercise, while for others, it is because of their diet. Certain nutrients strengthen bones, thus decreasing the chances of a fracture.

Usually, broken bones occur when performing day to day activities at home, work, or school. Some can be prevented while others cannot, but there are means of decreasing the possibility of fractures occurring. These are day to day preventative measures.

Physical Exercise

Bone strength will vary depending on the amount of exercise that one does. Muscles in the body usually become more extensive and more energetic after they have been used in the form of exercise. This principle applies to bones as well; the more one exercises their bone, the stronger and thicker they get. Bone exercise is usually determined by the ability of the bone to handle the weight of your body during physical activity.

Two forms of exercise are crucial in developing the density of bones, and they are as follows.

Weight-Bearing Physical Exercise

These forms of exercise usually involve movement in defiance of gravity while being in an upright position. There are two types of weight-bearing activities, and they are of high impact and low impact exercises. High impact exercises are those stress bones and joints. For example, jogging, running, dancing, aerobic exercises, skipping rope exercises, basketball, lacrosse, racquet, field hockey, soccer, gymnastics, climbing stairs or going back and forth a steep hill, hiking, tennis, and volleyball. Low impact exercises are better for those who may have difficulty in doing high impact exercises. Examples of low impact exercises cross-country ski machines, low impact aerobics, downhill & cross-country skiing, stair-step machines, and elliptical training machines. Some activities are healthy, but they don't lead to much bone-strengthening, such as cycling and swimming. It would be advisable for those who rely on swimming and cycling to include other forms of exercise in their routine, which will strengthen their bones. It is vital to go for a health check-up before beginning a new exercise regimen, especially where one does not exercise very often. The medical check-up will aid in establishing whether one is suffering from a medical complication such as high blood pressure, heart disease, or diabetes. Anyone beginning a new exercise program should take it slow in the beginning to allow for the body to adjust.

Muscle Bearing Physical Exercise

As the muscles strengthen, so do the bones, which in turn decreases the chances of a fracture occurring. Muscle exercises are done where one lifts a certain amount of weight against gravity, depending on their capabilities. A synonym to muscle bearing physical activity is resistance exercise. Examples of muscle-strengthening activities are as follows: use of weight machines such as bench pressing, exercises involving the use of elastic bands, lifting any kind of weight, for example, massive jugs filled with water and raising one's body weight. Using one's body weight is done a lot during yoga and Pilates, thus making them a type of muscle strengthening exercise. Yoga and Pilates require one to have balance; therefore, if one has a condition that they cannot risk a fall, so it would be advisable to avoid such exercises (or to limit) for anyone with balance issues. As mentioned earlier, some conditions affect the strength of bones, which means the person must very careful when exercising. An example would be people who have osteoporosis, and bones with minimal density should stay clear of specific positions that arise from certain forms of exercise. For example, people who have had fractures on their spine as a result of osteoporosis should avoid the following situations:

- Activities that require one to be in a far-reaching position.

- Bending forward could further hurt the spine

- Quick twisting movements

- Any physical exercise that would have a likelihood of a fall.

It is advisable for those who have osteoporosis to mostly do low impact weight-bearing exercises. Most of these exercises will not worsen a back fracture.

The Amount of Exercise

Bone strengthening goes hand in hand with practice, but the question that arises is the amount of exercise that should be done to yield results. The following are the exercise requirements of each form of exercise.

• Weight-Bearing Physical Activity

These types of exercises ought to be done for 3o minutes every single day for five or seven days in a week. One has the option of doing the exercise for 30 minutes consistently or do two sets of 15 minutes or three of 10 minutes. It doesn't matter which so long as it totals 3o minutes at the end of the day. An example would be having three sessions of weight-bearing exercises for 10 minutes, thus adding up to 30 minutes at the end of all the sessions. It does not matter whether one does the activity for 30 minutes or in breaks; the result of bone strength will be the same. One other means of ensuring one achieves the 30 minutes during the day would be by taking the stairs rather than the elevator or escalator, walking to work, or any other place and parking the vehicle further so that you walk more.

• Muscle-Strengthening Exercises

These forms of exercise ought to be done twice or thrice a week. One should identify one activity that would strengthen each muscle group adding up to 8 to 12 exercises. Each exercise should consist of one or two sets, which are repeated 8 or 10 times. An example would be lifting weight eight times in a row as one set will be a set made up of 8 repetitions. You can decrease the repetitions depending on the capabilities of their body and increase gradually as their muscles strengthen.

Where a person suffers from osteoporosis or has weak bones, it is recommended that they use light weights with 10 or 15 repetitions. It is also best to listen to your body. If you're in pain, stop doing what you're doing. Take it slowly, one step at a time. If you are limited with time, exercising one part of the body every other day, such as the arms on one day, the legs the next, etc. can be very helpful.

It is also important to note that it is very healthy to experience muscle soreness for a couple of days at the beginning of the exercise. If the pain lasts for a longer time you may be doing far much more than your body can handle and it would be advisable to slow down. It is recommended that in cases of fractures or osteoporosis, a physiotherapist should guide such an individual not to worsen the condition.

Three other forms of exercises are linked to bone strengthening. These include:

Balance Exercises

These forms of exercise focus on the leg bone strength, thus increasing your balance and reducing the chances of a fall. A reduction in the risk of a fall decreases the chances of a fracture occurring from a falling accident.

Posture Exercises

These forms of exercise lead to better posture and decrease sloping or rounded shoulders. A decrease in sloping or rounded shoulders also reduces the chances of a fracture on the spine occurs.

Functional Exercises

These forms of exercise increase the range of movement, which in turn aids one in day to day activities and lowers the chances of falling and fractures. A few examples where one should perform functional exercises would be where they struggle to get up from seats or going up the stairs.

Consumption of Foods that are Rich in Nutrients that Strengthen Bones

During the development stage of a child, nutrients are absorbed to promote their growth process. When the child grows into an adult, the nutrients are absorbed to maintain the body. For example, a child can consume calcium to enable the growth of their bones, but as an adult, the calcium will primarily be used for strengthening the bones.

Bones with low density tend to break easily. Consequently, these children and adults need to consume foods that are rich in nutrients to promote the strength of bones, thus limiting the occurrence of fractures.

Foods Rich in Calcium

Bones store calcium, which is essential for the development and strength of bones. The hormones within the body facilitate the movement of calcium to and from bones. A hormone referred to as parathyroid is responsible for a high calcium level within the blood. The basis is to control the calcium leaving the bones, which lower the density of the bones. Another hormone is calcitonin, which lowers calcium content in the bloodstream, thus ensuring that the calcium is stored within the bone. The reason why calcium may leave the bone is to aid muscle cells, which are crucial for many purposes, including heart function. The calcium level in the bones will depend on the amount the blood needs to perform other roles within the body. Foods that are rich in calcium can be found in vegetables. Calcium-rich foods lead to bones that have a high mass. The absence of consuming foods that are rich in calcium is beneficial to all age groups. Calcium leads to the avoidance of bone-related conditions such as osteoporosis which is common amongst older people.

The consumption of protein-rich foods is essential in the development of bones. 50% of bones are composed of protein. Bone breakdown and formation is affected by the amount of protein that one consumes. The absorption of calcium into the bones will be affected by the amount of protein that one consumes. Research has revealed that high consumption of protein leads to a lot of calcium leaving the bone as a means of reacting to the additional acid level of the blood. There is more research that has revealed that the consequence of high consumption of protein only affects those that consume over 100 grams a day. The diet should be balanced to prevent the occurrence of a high quantity of any nutrients in the body. Reports have revealed that older women have a high bone mass when they consume foods that are rich in protein. These women tend to have a decreased fracture occurrence rate of the bones on their hips, legs, arms, and spine. A concern arises between the possibility of weight gain from consuming foods that are rich in protein. This issue was addressed by the advice that those who are on a weight-loss regime have the option of consuming proteins that are low in calories.

Consumption of Foods that are Rich in Vitamin D

These two nutrients are vital in the development of bone. This leads to the formation of strong bones. The nutrient can both be found in different food types, but it can also be found to be sourced from the sun. Vitamin D aids in the absorption of calcium into the bones, which in turn helps in preventing bone-related diseases from occurring. Research has revealed that people who consume foods that are low on calcium tend to have low bone, thus increasing the likelihood of fractures. Vitamin D can be found from foods such as liver and cheese.

Chapter Fifteen

Medical Advancements

Medical Advancements in the Recovery of Bones: Fracture Repair Using Stem Cells

This is a method that has recently been established, but there is still research being conducted surrounding the procedure. The report has indicated that it may be a breakthrough in reducing the need for bone grafting in severe fractures. Over the years, a fracture that had difficulty healing would cause the need for bone transplant or any other type of surgery.

Currently, there is a possibility of a stem cell recovery method for broken bones. This treatment applies genes and stems cells as an effort to reduce the invasive nature of other procedures. Cedars- Sinai Medical Centre, which is located in Los Angeles, has a research team that would test stem cell therapy on animals. The research revealed that the cells would cause the tissue bones to regrow. Once the method has been approved as applicable and safe in human beings, then it will be the ideal method of repairing severely fractured bones, thus pushing out bone grafting.

The Skeletal Regeneration and Stem Cell therapy Program, which was established by the Department of Surgical and Cedars- Sinai Board of Governors Regenerative Medicine Institute, was impressed by the results. The Co-Director of the program, Dan Gazit, stated that the discovery of stem cells in the recovery of bone would be a huge advancement in orthopedics. The details of the research were documented and its contents published under the journal Science Translation Medicine.

The invasive nature of bone grafts, which involves the placement of bone within the fractured area of the body can be reduced by this latest discovery. The bones in bone grafting are usually sourced from a donor or within the body of the patient. One of the challenges associated with this method is the absence of a healthy bone that can be used in surgery and the complications that arise from the application of bone grafting.

The Method of Application of Stem Cells

The method is applied by placing a collagen matrix that consists of bone generation genes into the stem cells, thus promoting the repair of the cells. The collagen matrix is injected into the gap, which would be the fractured area for more than two weeks to yield results. There is an application of an ultrasound pulse and microbubbles to ensure that the collagen matrix is inserted into the cells. The stem cells are drawn from the body, as reported by Gadi Pelled. He is an Assistant Professor of Surgery located in Cedar Sinai Hospital and has had medical book publications over the years. The professor further stated that the method would be the efficient means of bone repair due to its injectable nature rather than the surgical method. The research revealed that the fractures would take up nearly 8 weeks to recover after the procedure was initialized. The healing of the bone that underwent this method would be just as strong as one that had undergone bone grafting surgery. Dan Gazit revealed that this method of bone healing was the most ideal and would be preferred in comparison to the bone graft method. The doctor further stated that the pain that usually follows from the retrieval of the bone through surgery would be avoided by the application of this method. The infection rate that is associated with surgeries will decrease in the case of fractures because this method is not invasive.

The method would also be suited for fractures that have resulted in huge gaps between the bones, which are usually very difficult to heal. There would be a need for multiple injections in cases involving large gaps to increase the amount of bone that could grow. Reports have revealed that this method would be the most ideal in cases where the bone has difficulty healing after a long time. However, there is still some research that has to be conducted before the method can be approved for use amongst human beings. The stem cell method is not exactly new in the medical field, but after years of research, the method has significantly improved. The current method has been proven to be the breakthrough in broken bone recovery.

The Concerns Associated with Stem Cell Recovery

The method sounds ideal because it relies on the stem cells that are generated by the body leading to a decrease that is usually associated with other forms of treatment. Nevertheless, some concerns are raised regarding the safety of the procedure. The method must be proven to be safe for human use, for example, by establishing that the method is non-toxic. These are one of the concerns that were raised by Dr. Zulma Gazit, the co-director of the Skeletal Regeneration and Stem Cell Therapy Program who works in the Department of Surgical and Cedars- Sinai Board of Governors Regenerative Medicine Institute.

Medical Advancements in the Health Sector: Affordable Care Act and its Impact on Nursing Practice

The Affordable Care Act led to an increase in the number of patients landing in the hospital, which increased the role of the nurse as a primary caregiver. The surge in the number of patients is because the legislation provides for health insurance coverage for every American citizen. There were severe medical emergencies such as the fracture of a skull or open fractures to which some people did not have medical assistance. Subsequently, after the enactment of the Affordable Care Act, there was an increase in the number of fracture-related cases in the emergency care unit. The increase was a result of the people who could not access healthcare in the past due to various factors such as finance, discrimination, and inequality, amongst others. As earlier explained, one of the challenges of the administration of emergency care is inaccessibility to specific groups of people within the community. This makes it easier for patients who have experienced fractures to have access to the emergency care unit immediately.

Quality Measures and Pay for Performance

Pay for performance is a principle that provides financial incentives to healthcare providers depending on their healthcare delivery. The rationale behind the principle is that healthcare quality will significantly improve in the presence of monetary persuasion of healthcare providers. This was a positive principle in the provision of emergency care, thereby assistant patients that suffer from fractures. The quality of treatment provided was significantly higher due to the monetary attachment placed. The components that measure quality include the following concerning the roles of nurses;

The Experience of Delivery of The Medical Care

The patient should have a smooth experience during the delivery of healthcare services. These health services also pertain to those that are delivered during fractured bone situations. The nurses should be caring and reassuring to the patient during their stay at the hospital. Cases that involve fractures are usually very intense, and the health providers need to reassure the patient and their family members. The cases are even more stressful when the patient is a child. This act will ensure that the patient is the primary focus while they are at the hospital, which will further lead to their comfort.

The Medical Outcome

This quality of healthcare pertains to the result of the healthcare provided by the medical personnel. In the case of nurses, there are various means of measuring the outcomes. A few examples include delivering medication to the patient, monitoring patients in the recovery room, communicating with the patient regarding their discharge, and the care given to the patient during their admission, amongst others. The outcome of the patient is also associated with the recovery rate from the fracture and whether the patient has recovered with a deformity or is capable of performing their daily activities. The nurse has the role of monitoring the patient's vital signs to ensure that they are stable while at the hospital. The instability of the patient could be associated with the possibility of a clot infection after bone repair surgery. The health providers should, therefore, keep a close eye on the patient. This measure of quality would establish the monetary reward that a nurse deserves.

Process of Care

This quality measure looks into the process of delivery of healthcare. This measure aims to ensure that while the patient is within the hospital's care, they do not acquire complications arising from the standards of care delivered. An example would be a nurse, ensuring that the patient does not acquire an infection linked to the quality of healthcare provided. The quality of the process of care requires a nurse to immediately attending to the patient whenever they are in need. The nurse must also inform the doctor of any significant changes in the vitals of the patient. These are the actions that ensure high quality in the process of healthcare delivery.

Provision of Primary Care

Nurses are the primary healthcare providers in a health care system. Primary healthcare is the medical care provided at the initial stage when a patient lands in the hospital. For example, a patient with a fracture should immediately be attended to by a medical officer as soon as the patient arrives in the hospital. The nurse must take in the patient and provide all the essential medical necessities before the doctor's arrival.

The nursing profession has undergone several transformations which have increased their role in the health sector.

Nursing Staff

Reports have indicated that nurses can significantly affect the quality of healthcare delivered to the people due to their vital role in healthcare. Nurses are crucial in ensuring that there are no medical mistakes in the healthcare system and that there is the management of patients admitted to the hospital. Research has established that increasing the nurses' responsibility in managing infections would remarkably decrease the infection rate of patients. Nurses also ensure that the patient's experience while at the hospital is comfortable, thus making the adaptation to the environment much more manageable.

Department of Veterans Affairs

The United States Department of Veterans Affairs has progressively increased the roles that nurses play in the healthcare system, which has had notable results. This is beneficial to military officers that encounter fractures while in service. There is a need for emergency care to be transmitted in such situations. The expanded roles of nurses in management and leadership have led to a more accessible and high-quality healthcare system.

The Role of Nurses and The Needs of The Patient

The safety of the patient has become the most critical factor in the delivery of healthcare. The roles of nurses have evolved to being centered around the needs of the patients. The patient's comfort is the nurse's main objective, which must be reflected in the hospital's agenda. A nurse ensures that the patient is assisted with daily activities such as showering or eating whenever they lack the capability. Fractures result in limited mobility, and such patients need the assistance of nurses. This act ensures that the patient feels comfortable the entire time while at the hospital.

Geisinger Health System of Pennsylvania provides for comprehensive healthcare for millions of people at a much higher quality than other healthcare systems. The reason behind this success is because the system is more focused on the needs of the patients.

The Escalating Use of Telehealth

Telehealth is the means a patient can use with the aid of technology to access medical care from doctors or nurses. This method has led to the roles of nurses expanding with the application of telehealth in the hospital. A patient can access a healthcare provider through phone calls, video calls, remote monitoring, and other technological means of communication. This can be crucial in the delivery of medical services in the case where a broken bone as occurred. The American Hospital Association has revealed that seventy-six percent of hospitals in the United States have inculcated telehealth in the healthcare delivery system. Nurses in much more advanced hospitals in the urban areas would have a consultancy role in educating the nurses in the rural sector through telehealth in the form of video calls.

Increased Specialization

General nurses are losing demand in the healthcare system due to the need for specialized nurses. These are nurses that have dedicated to one medical field rather than having general medical competence. Some nurses are specialized in the orthopedic field, thereby rendering their services invaluable to patients that are suffering from a bone fracture. This qualification assures the hospital that a nurse is extremely competent in a specific area, allocating them to that medical department. Consequently, nurses have a role in ensuring that they acquire expertise in one area to ensure that they deliver quality healthcare.

Conclusion

In conclusion, emergency care is a very serious issue that would benefit a lot of people. The steps mentioned in this book are crucial, and one misstep could cost the victim far much more than anticipated. It is, therefore, important for people to have the emergency care basics in cases of a medical emergency, giving them the knowledge and ability to manage a broken bone.

An infringement on the right to health is an infringement on the right to life. The ethical perspective is that many laws have been drawn from the fundamental virtues of human beings, such as the protection of human life, thus giving birth to the right to health. Legal validation for the need for emergency care systems pushes states to put in place measures that guarantee the protection of human life. Some bone fractures are deadly, and there is a need for an emergency care system to manage them.

Severe fractures usually take much longer to heal and require much more invasive procedures such as bone grafting. Another invasive procedure is open reduction and internal fixation surgery, which is typically a surgical procedure using pins, rods, and metal screws to repair the broken bone. Less severe fractures are usually treated with a cast to align the bone and enhance healing of the broken area. Certain actions must take place after surgery, such as the placing of ice on the healing bone and the elevation of the broken bone to reduce swelling. After surgery, the patient should consume foods with vitamin C and D to ensure that the bone heals faster.

Some people have lived their whole lives without ever breaking a bone in their body. This disparity can be attributed to luck and significant genes for some people, exercise, for others, and maybe a healthy diet for some. Certain nutrients strengthen bones, thus decreasing the chances of a fracture.

Bone strength will vary depending on the amount of exercise that one does. Muscles in the body usually become more extensive and more energetic after they have been used in the form of exercise. This principle applies to bones as well; the more one exercises their bone, the stronger and thicker they get. Bone exercise is usually determined by the ability of the bone to handle the weight of your body during physical activity. Due to the difference in the type of fractures, there are situations where a fractured bone will not heal on its own, or the healed bone will result in a deformity. This kind of recovery may force a person to consider other means of recovery, such as bone grafting or a knee replacement surgery. Bone grafting is also known as a bone transplant. As the name suggests, it is how a surgeon will obtain a bone from a donor or within the body of the patient and transfer it to the fractured area. The technicality of the procedure has its risks, such as the possibility of the body rejecting the bone graft. Knee replacement surgery is when an artificial knee referred to as a prosthesis is placed in the fractured area within the knee.

There is an advancement in the medical sector in terms of the quality of healthcare being provided. This will benefit a lot of people that suffer from fractures and require medical assistance. They are several principles that have arisen to increase quality to which this book discusses. One of these principles is the measure of outcome. This quality of healthcare pertains to the result of the healthcare provided by the medical personnel. In the case of nurses, there are various means of measuring the outcomes A few examples include delivering medication to the patient, monitoring patients in the recovery room, communicating with the patient regarding their discharge. The care given to the patient during their admission, amongst others, the outcome of the patient is also associated with the recovery rate from the fracture and whether the patient has recovered with a deformity or is capable of performing their daily activities

The nurse has the role of monitoring the patient's vital to ensure that they are stable while at the hospital. The instability of the patient could be associated with the possibility of a clot infection after bone repair surgery. The health providers should, therefore, keep a close eye on the patient. This measure of quality would establish the monetary reward that a nurse deserves. Another principle that was established was the process of care. The principle is an aspect of the quality measure that looks into the process of delivery of healthcare. This measure aims to ensure that while the patient is within the hospital's care, they do not acquire complications arising from the standards of care delivered. An example would be a nurse, ensuring that the patient does not acquire an infection linked to the quality of healthcare provided as we shall soon establish, infection is one of the risks associated with bone repair surgery. The quality of the process of care requires a nurse to immediately attending to the patient whenever they are in need. The nurse must also inform the doctor of any significant changes in the vitals of the patient. These are the actions that ensure high quality in the process of healthcare delivery.

Conclusively, human rights are the cornerstone of the civilization of human beings, and in the case where a right has been provided for, the state must enforce it in cases of violation. Accordingly, it is important for institutions such as schools, hospitals, among others, to impart knowledge on emergency care, thus ensuring that most people can take care of each other in situations involving a broken bone.

If a broken bone occurs, you are now equipped to identify the type of fracture, assess the seriousness of the situation, and how to take first aid measures. Remember to always call 911 if there is any doubt as to the extent of an injury. Never put yourself in harm's way in an attempt to rescue another person. With the advice in this book, you should be equipped with the knowledge of how to attend to broken bones, what to expect once you arrive at the hospital, and the treatment options available.

Bibliography

Wessells, N. K., 1977. Tissue Interactions and Development. Menlo Park, CA, < https://onesearch.nihlibrary.ors.nih.gov/discovery/fulldispla y?vid=01NIH_INST:NIH&search_scope=NIHAll&tab=NI HCampus&docid=alma991000136649704686&lang=en&co ntext=L&adaptor=Local%20Search%20Engine&query=sub, exact,Fetus%20--%20Physiology,AND&mode=advanced

Kristen Fischer, 'Using Stem Cells to Heal Broken Bones' (Healthline, 13th June 2017) < https://www.healthline.com/health/bone-graft

Brian Krans, 'Bone Graft' (Healthline, November 2018) < https://www.healthline.com/health/bone-graft

Birk A.W., Bassuk E.L. (1984) The Concept of Emergency Care. In: Bassuk E.L., Birk A.W. (eds) Emergency Psychiatry. Critical Issues in Psychiatry (An Educational Series for Residents and Clinicians). Springer, Boston, MA < https://link.springer.com/chapter/10.1007/978-1-4684-4751-4_1

Hall, Brian K. "The Embryonic Development of Bone." American Scientist, vol. 76, no. 2, 1988, pp. 174–181. JSTOR,< file:///C:/Users/thela/Downloads/embryonicdevelofbone198 8%20(1).pdf

Antoinette Baujard 'Utilitarianism and Anti-Utilitarianism' (2013), page 3 <file:///C:/Users/thela/Downloads/Documents/1332.pdf

Healthline Editorial Team 'Bone Fracture Repair'/ (Healthline, 16th September 2018) < https://www.healthline.com/health/bone-graft

Julianne Schaeffer 'Blood Clot' (Healthline, 26th March 2016) < https://www.healthline.com/health/bone-graft

Levin L, Schwartz-Arad D. The effect of cigarette smoking on dental implants and related surgery. Implant Dent. 2005;14(4):357-361. < https://pubmed.ncbi.nlm.nih.gov/16361886

Linda Hepler 'First Aid for Broken Bones and Fractures' (Healthline, 8th July 2017) < https://www.healthline.com/health/bone-graft

Healthbeat 'Strength training builds more than muscles' (Harvard Health Publishing: Harvard Medical School) <https://www.health.harvard.edu/staying-healthy/strength-training-builds-more-than-muscles

National Osteoporosis Foundation "Exercise for your bone" (2013) < https://cdn.nof.org/wp-content/uploads/2016/02/Exercise-for-Your-Bone-Health.pdf

Benjamin Wedro, 'Broken Bone (Types of Bone Fractures)' (MedicineNet 2020) < https://www.medicinenet.com/broken_bone_types_of_bone_fractures/article.htm

Walsh SSM, Jarvis SN, Towner, et al. 'Annual incidence of unintentional injury among 54 000 children.' Inj Prev, 1996;2:16–20. <

https://injuryprevention.bmj.com/content/2/1/16.citation-tools

Gallagher SS, Finison K, Guyer B, et al. 'The incidence of injuries among 87 000 Massachusetts children and adolescents: results of the 1980–1981 statewide childhood injury prevention program surveillance system.' Am J Public Health, 1984;74:1340–7 < https://ajph.aphapublications.org/doi/abs/10.2105/AJPH.74.12.1340

Gerke R. 'How to Treat Fractures in the Wilderness.' Outdoor Survival Guide <http://www.theoutdoorsurvivalguide.com/fractures.html

Rivara FP, Calonge N, Thompson RS. 'Population-based study of unintentional injury incidence and impact during childhood.' Am J Public Health, 1989; 79:990–994. < https://ajph.aphapublications.org/doi/abs/10.2105/AJPH.79.8.990

Scheidt PC, Harel Y, Trumble AC, et al. 'The epidemiology of nonfatal injuries among US children and youth.' Am J Public Health, 1995; 85:932–938. < https://ajph.aphapublications.org/doi/abs/10.2105/AJPH.85.7.932

Walsh SS, Jarvis SN. 'Measuring the frequency of "severe" accidental injury in childhood.' J Epidemiol Community Health 1992; 46:26–32. < https://injuryprevention.bmj.com/content/4/3/194#ref-4

Rivara FP, Thompson RS, Thompson DC, and Calonge N. 'Injuries to children and adolescents: impact on physical health.' Pediatrics 1991;88: 783–788 < https://pediatrics.aappublications.org/content/88/4/783

United Nations Human Rights Office of the High Commissioner, 'Human Rights of Persons with disabilities https://www.ohchr.org/en/issues/disability/pages/disabilityindex.aspx

International Labour Organization 'Inclusion of People with Disabilities in Kenya' (2009).<http://www.ilo.org/wcmsp5/groups/public/---ed_emp/--ifp_skills/documents/publication/wcms_115097.pdf

Kenya National Population Census Report, 2009.<http://www.knbs.or.ke/Census%20Results/Presentation%20by%20Minister%20for%20Planning%20revised.pdf

World Health Organisation and The World Bank, 'World Report on Disability' (2011) page 29

Kenya National Survey for Persons with Disabilities <file:///C:/Users/thela/Downloads/Documents/KNSPWD-Main-Report.pdf

Reproductive Rights Movement' 2017 <file:///C:/Users/thela/Downloads/Documents/Disability-Briefing-Paper-FINAL.pdf

'Ensuring Equal Access To Health Services' (UM), <http://kenya.um.dk/en/danida-en/gender/ensuring-equal-access-to-health-services

<https://www.kenyaplex.com/resources/13450-challenges-faced-by-children-with-disability-in-kenya.asp

(Hrlibrary.umn.edu)<http://hrlibrary.umn.edu/edumat/hreduseries/TB6/pdfs/HRYes%20-%20Part%202%20-%20Chapter%208.pdf

'Challenges Faced By Disabled Persons And How The Government Can Intervene' (Bulawayo24 News, 2017) <https://bulawayo24.com/index-id-opinion-sc-columnist-byo-104288.html

Barker M, Power C, Roberts I. 'Injuries and the risk of disability in teenagers and young adults.' Arch Dis Child 1996; 75:156–8 < https://adc.bmj.com/content/75/2/156.abstractAbstract/FREE Full TextGoogle Scholar

Kopjar B, Wickizer TM. 'Fractures among children: incidence and impact on daily activities.' Injury Prevention 1998;4:194-197 < https://injuryprevention.bmj.com/content/4/3/194#ref-4

Institute of Medicine (US) Committee (2011). The Future of Nursing: Leading Change, Advancing Health. Washington (DC). National Academies Press (US). Retrieved from https://www.ncbi.nlm.nih.gov/books/NBK209871/

Purdue University Global. (2019). Top 10 Nursing Trends for 2020. Purdue University Global. Retrieved from https://www.purdueglobal.edu/blog/nursing/top-10-nursing-trends

Salmond, S. W, & Echevarria, M. (2017). Healthcare Transformation and Changing Roles for Nursing. Orthopedic nursing, 36(1), 12–25. Retrieved from https://www.ncbi.nlm.nih.gov/pmc/articles/PMC5266427/

EMERGENCY CARE

FOR BEGINNERS

How to Heal Someone Who Has Been Shot

BRANDA NURT

Introduction

W e live in a world where the escalation of violence can lead to terrifying outcomes. Firearms are dangerous weapons. The potential harm from a gunshot wound is a treat to be reckoned with, and for a good reason. These are potentially lethal wounds, and if we're not careful, they can take away our lives and the life of those close to us. In a world where firearms are increasingly easy to get, the risk of getting shot is higher than ever.

We can avoid dangerous neighborhoods and risky situations as a general rule; however, that doesn't guarantee we're safe from firearms. There's no completely safe place. If by any chance, you happen to be in the line of fire, it's better to be prepared than to let yourself be consumed by panic in your ignorance. In the face of trauma, time is of the essence. Receiving adequate treatment just after the gunshot wound dramatically increases the chance of survival and recovery. Your knowledge and proficiency can be the difference between life and death.

If you're reading this book, that means you're worried about the many situations in which you could face a gunshot wound without immediate medical assistance. You'll learn how to treat these injuries even if you have no professional health training at all. This knowledge is about the treatment someone should receive while waiting for an ambulance, but it's not limited to it. If you find yourself on a hunting trip, far away from civilization, it's better to be prepared to treat these wounds. The same could happen during natural disasters or any other circumstance where professional help isn't available. You'll become the caregiver needed in these circumstances. You'll learn how to save lives.

This book is organized to help you face these circumstances. The first chapter is a step-by-step explanation of what to do with a gunshot wound. It's oversimplified to help you as a reminder whenever the time comes. Or to have someone guide you with the book while you perform the treatment. This chapter is a condensation of all the knowledge presented here and should be kept on hand at all times. Starting with the second chapter, the rest of the book will teach you the basic knowledge behind the treatment techniques you must apply and an overall understanding of how the body functions. This chapter is where your journey truly starts. After you've read the rest of the book, the steps presented in the first chapter will be much easier for you to understand; and when you follow them to treat someone, you'll know exactly how to do it and why you're doing it.

Don't ever feel discouraged if you're not a professional. Some people cower down in the face of an emergency while others understand that, in dire circumstances, there aren't wasted efforts. It's better to do your best even if it's not enough than to live with the regret of knowing you could've at least done something. If you're reading this book, you're already committed to helping others and saving lives if you must. Take this knowledge seriously, practice the techniques at home, and build your first aid kit according to his book's recommendations. If the time comes, you'll be ready to save lives.

Note: If you're in a life-threatening or emergency medical situation, seek medical assistance immediately.

Chapter 1

Facing the Emergency

Here's the fast walkthrough of what everyone should follow to heal a gunshot wounded patient. Follow these steps until professional paramedics get to the patient and can take over the treatment. If there's no chance of paramedics reaching the patient, follow these steps until the patient's ready to be transported to a suitable health center.

Step 1: Scream for Help and Assess the Situation

The first thing you must do with any traumatized patients is to call for help. Ask for those around you to call the authorities (call 911) and make sure they're on their way while dealing with the patient. Ask for help getting your first aid kit ready or gathering first aid supplies from those around you. You will need:

- An automatic external defibrillator

- Blood pressure monitor

- Tourniquets

- Scissors

- Compression bandages

- Chest seal

- Space blanket

- Combat gauze

- Nasopharyngeal tube

- Lubricant

- Surgical tape

- Splints

- Cervical collar

- Prepared syringes with epinephrine and atropine

- As many gauze bandages as you can gather

- At least two pairs of gloves.

Also, make a quick assessment of the situation surrounding the patient. If neither you nor the patient is safe where you are, it's imperative to take the patient to a safe place before starting his treatment.

Step 2: Check for Breathing and Pulse/Run Triage

If the patient's unconscious, make sure that he's breathing by placing your hand under his nose and watching his chest's movements. Then check if he has a pulse by placing your index, middle, and ring finger over the right side of his right wrist, right under the palm (more details in chapter seven). If you can't feel his pulse, place your head over his chest to listen to his heartbeat. If his heart's not beating and/or he's not breathing, jump to step 10. If he's breathing and his heart is beating, move on to the next step. If there's a mass casualty with many gunshot wound patients, prioritize patients – those with severe bleeding and who seem to be in a bad way but are still breathing and those who are no longer breathing and have no pulse or heartbeat (more details in chapter eight).

Step 3: Discover the Body to Search for Wounds

Bullets can:

- Penetrate the body and stay there (handgun)

- Pierce the body in a straight line by entering from one side and leaving through the other side (more powerful weapons)

- Penetrate the body, impact on a bone, and rebound. The bullet may stay there after deviating or exit from another part of the body.

Search for these wounds and locate them. Use scissors or blades to cut through the patient's clothing and get easy access to the injuries.

Put on a pair of gloves if you have them available or as soon as possible to follow the steps.

Step 4: Identify Massive Hemorrhages and Stop Them

Wounds losing a large amount of blood and wounds with red and bright blood shooting out in short bursts are the ones you must address first (more details in chapter 9).

Lift the Wounds

If the wounds are located on any of the limbs, lift these limbs above heart-level and keep them there. Be careful not to move or rotate the neck or the torso and not to lift healthy extremities.

Apply Pressure

Use gauze bandages to apply pressure directly over the bleeding wounds. Use your palms and the strength of your arms to apply the pressure. Do these with all massive bleedings prioritizing those from the neck, torso, and extremities in that order. Don't apply pressure to nose bleeding or bleeding through the ears. Use combat gauzes on neck wounds if you have them available.

Pack the Wound

A wound located on the limbs or the torso must be filled with gauze bandages until it's sealed. Try to fit the first gauze in the direction of the patient's head. If you have combat gauze available, use these as the first gauze bandages. Don't take out the bandages once they're in place. Don't do this on wounds located on the neck.

Apply a Compression Bandage

Once you've packed the wound with gauze bandages, use compression bandages to fix these gauze bandages in place. Make sure it's tight enough to keep the pressure and tie them well enough to keep them from disarming. Don't do this on wounds located on the neck.

Use a Tourniquet

This is just for uncontrolled bleeding in limbs. If you have a commercial tourniquet available, use this one or two inches over the wound and strap it on tight enough to make it uncomfortable for the patient and stop the bleeding. If you don't have a commercial tourniquet available, create an improvised tourniquet using a compression bandage, rope, tie, belt, or anything you can use to squeeze the limb hard enough. If you lack the strength to squeeze the improvised tourniquet, tie a stick or anything you can use as a lever over the tourniquet and twist it until you get the desired effect. Tourniquets should not be placed over joints or left in place for longer than two hours.

Step 5: Assess the Airway

If the patient's ability to speak, cry or yell, he's able to breathe. If he's unconscious or you're not sure, start by checking the windpipe to make sure it's not damaged or obstructed. Carefully and slowly tilt the head back and lift the patient's chin to facilitate breathing. If the patient's not breathing, jump to step 10.

Step 6: Assess Breathing

Check the patient's thorax to see how he's breathing (more details in chapter nine); look for an asymmetrical thorax or any other anomalies. Evaluate respiratory rate by counting how many breaths does the patient takes for twenty seconds and multiplying that by three (more details in chapter seven); if the patient's not breathing, jump towards step 10.

Check the torso front and back from the shoulders to the belly button, searching for penetrating wounds; make sure not to flex, extend, or rotate the neck while searching in the patient's back. If there's a penetrating wound anywhere from the shoulders to the belly button, place a chest seal over it and seal it shut by using surgical tape (or industrial tape) in three out of the four edges of the seal. If there's no chest seal available, use anything hard enough, such as foil or a credit card. Check after three minutes if the patient's respiratory condition has improved or gotten worse. If the situation has improved, leave the chest seal; if it has gotten worse, remove the chest seal.

Step 7: Assess Circulation

Measure the patient's blood pressure with the help of an automatic blood pressure monitor if you have one available. If the systolic blood pressure is under ninety and/or the pulse rate is below fifty, that means the patient is in bad condition. If the patient's in bad shape, or if he's deteriorating rapidly in that direction, check for untreated bleeding wounds or reassess the wounds you've treated to ensure no massive hemorrhages are deteriorating the patient's condition (more details in chapter nine).Begin by taking the patient's pulse rate and blood pressure (more details in chapter seven). Using your index, middle, and ring finger, feel the patient's pulse under the palm of his hand, count the number of pulses and multiply them by four to get the pulse rate. M

Step 8: Assess Head Injuries and Treat Hypothermia

Check for head injuries and immobilize the cervical spine if you suspect head and/or (more details in chapter six). Strap a cervical collar around the neck if you have one available. If you don't have one available, make an improvised immobilizer using a pair of hats, a pair of shoes, small pillows, or even cardboard. Tie these around the neck with a compression bandage, a belt, shoelaces, or anything available. To place these objects around the neck, lift the head and the shoulders of the patient *while making sure you don't flex, extend, or rotate the neck* by any means. Make sure not to tie the immobilizer so tight that it obstructs airflow or circulation. Once you've finished with the immobilization of the cervical spine, check the Glasgow Coma Scale to assess the degree of possible brain trauma/damage (more details in chapter seven):

Glasgow	Coma	Scale
Eyes	Open spontaneously	+4
	Open to sound (speak to the patient to assess)	+3
	Open to pressure (squeeze fingertips to assess)	+2
	Don't open (squeeze fingertips to assess)	+1
Verbal	Oriented (can remember time, place, and name)	+5
	Confused (can't remember time, place, and/or name)	+4
	Inappropriate words (speech doesn't make sense)	+3
	Incomprehensible sounds (unable to mouth words)	+2
	No verbal response (squeeze fingertips to assess)	+1
Motor	Obey commands (speak to assess)	+6

	Localize pain (pinch zone between shoulder and neck to assess)	+5
	Normal flexion (squeeze fingertips to assess if he flexes the elbow and withdraws the hand without taking it to his body)	+4
	Abnormal flexion (squeeze fingertips to assess if he flexes the elbow and withdraws the hand by placing it over his body)	+3
	Extension to pain (squeeze fingertips to assess if he extends the elbow)	+2
	No motor response (squeeze fingertips to assess)	+1

Add the points from the three main aspects to get a reading of the GCC.

To avoid hypothermia, place a space blanket over the patient's body. If no space blanket is available, use a wool blanket, coats, or anything else that may provide warmth.

Step 9: Check Other Wounds, Immobilize, and Prepare for Transportation

Start by treating wounds that aren't bleeding as much. Remember, massive bleeding was addressed in step Four. Apply pressure over the wounds with gauze bandages, apply wound packing if the wounds are not in the neck, and secure them with compression wounds (more details in chapter nine).

Immobilizations

Apply an immobilization whenever you believe there may be a fracture (more details in chapter six). If you suspect arm, forearm, wrist, or hand fracture, use a splint to immobilize the affected limb. If you don't have a commercial splint available, use a plank, a stick, cardboard, or anything else hard enough and able to adapt to the arm's shape to immobilize the affected segment by securing it with a compression bandage. If possible, make sure that the splint can immobilize the proximal and the distal joint of the affected segment. The elbow must be immobilized in flexion of ninety degrees. If there's no splint able to immobilize the elbow or the shoulder, use a sling to immobilize these joints.

Use a triangular bandage if available to make an arm sling if you suspect ribs, clavicle, shoulder, or an upper arm fracture. Place the triangular bandage under the arm with the forearm placed horizontally over the patient's body, and the patient's elbow flexed at a ninety degrees angle. Take the higher tip of the bandage to the healthy shoulder and behind the neck to reach the affected shoulder. Take the other tip of the bandage over the forearm and towards the affected shoulder and tie it to the other tip to finish the sling.

Use a triangular bandage if available to make an elevated arm sling if you suspect forearm, wrist, or hand fracture; also, to stop forearm or hand bleeding. Place the patient's injured forearm diagonally over his chest with the fingertips over his healthy shoulder. Then place the triangular bandage over the patient's forearm with one tip over the injured hand. Tuck the lower edge of the bandage under the patient's forearm and elbow. Get the other end of the bandage behind the patient's back and elevate it diagonally until it meets with the first end of the bandage. Tie both ends together to finish the elevated arm sling.

If there's no triangular bandage available, use a compression bandage, belt, or folded cloth to make a collar-and-cuff sling. Take the center of the compression bandage behind the patient's neck, with both ends over his body pointing towards his feet. Get his forearm in position (horizontal for upper arm injuries and elevated for lower arm injuries). Once the forearm is in place, get both ends of the compression bandage to tie a knot over the wrist, take the ends around the wrist, and tie a second knot below the wrist to finish the collar-and-cuff sling. Remember to be careful not to change the neck's position during the application of the sling.

Legs immobilizations work only with splints. If you suspect leg fracture, use a commercial splint on the affected area of the leg to immobilize it; the splint should immobilize the affected segment's proximal and distal joints. The ankle must be flexed in ninety degrees, and the knee should be slightly flexed; placing a roll of bandage under the joint can give the knee the desired degree of flexion. If there's no commercial splint available, create an improvised splint using planks, cardboard, or any suitable materials and tie it with a compression bandage. If there are no appropriate materials, it's acceptable to use the healthy leg as a splint for the affected leg.

NOTE: After the immobilization of the arm or leg is completed, squeeze the fingertips of the immobilized limb. If they recover their color in less than three seconds, their circulation isn't compromised. If they don't recover their color in less than three seconds, their circulation may be compromised, and the immobilization should be loosened.

Thoracic and lumbar spine immobilization can only be done with a stretcher and should be left to the professional paramedics. If no paramedics are coming, and the patient is to be transported to a health center, thoracic and lumbar spine immobilization must be achieved as possible by carrying the patient in a group while avoiding torso flexion, extension, and rotation.

Receiving the Paramedics

When the paramedics take over the patient's treatment, you must notify them of the information you gathered, the treatment techniques you applied, and the vital signs and other assessments to make their job easier.

Choosing a Health Center for Transportation

If you're the one who'll take charge of the transportation, it's crucial to get the patient to a suitable health center (more details in chapters seven and eight). A patient with a Glasgow Coma Scale score below fourteen points, a respiratory rate below 10 or above 29, and/or a systolic blood pressure under 90 mmHg must be transported to a trauma center. Patients with penetrating wounds to the head, neck, torso, or extremities proximal to the elbows or knees, thorax deformities or instability, pelvic or skull fractures, paralysis, or a pulseless extremity must also be taken to a trauma center. The rest of the patients could be transported to any health center available.

Step 10: Practice CPR

A patient with cardiopulmonary arrest needs Cardiopulmonary Resuscitation or CPR as soon as possible (more details in chapter five).

Compressions

Make sure the patient is over a hard and flat surface and kneel beside the patient's shoulder. Press the heel of one of your hands over the patient's sternum at nipple height, place your second hand over the first hand, and lean over the patient to align your shoulders with your hands. Press down over the patient's chest at 100 to 120 compressions per minute using the weight of your upper body. Make sure you're pressing down at least 2 inches, but less than 2.4 inches. Do this until you've completed 30 chest compressions.

Airway

Carefully tilt the patient's head back and lift his chin to open the airway.

Breathing

Close the patient's nose with your fingers, take the air, place your mouth over the patient's mouth to create a seal, and let the air into the patient's mouth during one second. Check to see if the patient's chest rises; if it does, the rescue breath was provided correctly. If the chest doesn't rise, make the face-tilt and chin-lift maneuver again and try it one more time. If the abdomen is the one that grows, you're blowing too hard. Provide two rescue breaths to complete a CPR cycle.

AED

If an automatic external defibrillator is available, follow the instructions and keep repeating CPR cycles until the patient starts breathing again or the paramedics arrive. If there's no AED available, keep doing the CPR cycles until the patient starts breathing again or the paramedics arrive.

Respiratory Arrest

If the patient doesn't breathe, but his heart keeps beating, all he needs is the breathing part of the CPR. Give one rescue breath every 5-6 seconds until he starts breathing again, or the patient can receive professional help.

Going Back to the Scheme of Treatment

Once the patient's heart starts beating once again, and his breathing resumes, return to the treatment step you were in before you jumped to the tenth step and resume the step-by-step treatment from there.

Note: If you're in a life-threatening or emergency medical situation, seek medical assistance immediately.

Chapter 2

Anatomical Considerations

The treatment of any injured patient requires extensive knowledge of the anatomical structures of the body, especially those that are vulnerable and vital. Before you learn how to study a patient from head to toe, first you must understand what you're looking for. Some injuries are more important and critical than others because of the associated structures, and it's impossible to understand this unless you develop a deep knowledge of the human body. In this chapter, we're going to allow you to understand the body's anatomy on a very basic level. We'll prioritize the essential knowledge to understand the possible consequences of a gunshot wound, and how to deal with them.

Localization

The study of the human body is extensive, and it can get confusing. You can't say that your index finger is at the left side of your thumb because that would only be true for your right hand when the palm is facing front, or your left hand when the palm is facing back. This means that terminology such as "left" and "right" can't be used to describe the anatomy of the human body accurately. A universal language has been created to describe and understand anatomy without confusion, as well as a standard body position in which anatomy is described.

The anatomical position is the standard situation of any bodies studied in anatomy. This is described with the body straight up, facing the observer, with both feet planted on the ground facing onward, and both arms at the sides, with palms facing forward. This means that the thumbs of the hands will be pointing "outwards," and the inner sides of the biceps will be facing inwards since the arms will be slightly rotated in this position. The anatomical position looks similar to this picture.

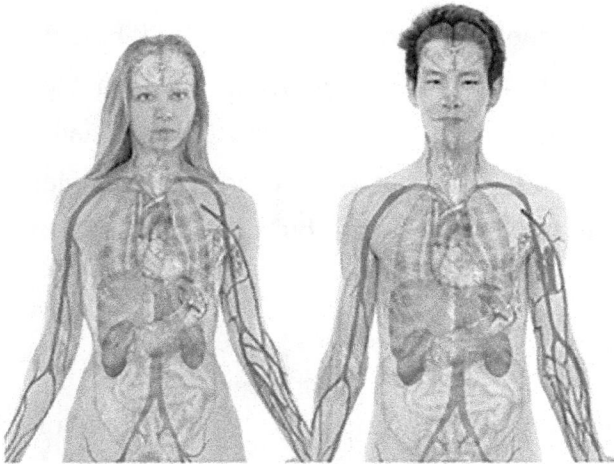

http://commons.wikimedia.org/wiki/File:Female_with_organs.png
http://commons.wikimedia.org/wiki/File:Male_with_organs.png

Every time you see an anatomy 3D model, chances are that the model will assume this position, so you'll get used to it in no time.

319

Then you have the different terms used to describe the location of any part of the human body. These are also universal, and you'll find them in any anatomy book.

Anterior means near the front of the body, and posterior means that it's located towards the back of the body. Midline is the imaginary vertical line that divides the body between right and left. Medial is closer to the vertical midline, and lateral is something that's further from the vertical midline. Superior and inferior are just what you'd expect, something that's located upwards versus something that's rather downwards. Proximal and distal are similar, but these terms are related to the origin of a structure. So proximal is closer to the structure's origin, and distal is further from its origin. Therefore, for example, your elbow will be proximal from your forearm, because it's closer to the shoulder, and your fingertips will be distal from your forearm because they're further from your shoulder. Finally, superficial means closer to the surface (the skin) and deep means closer to your body's interior (your heart, for example). Once you learn and understand these terms, you're ready to start learning about basic human anatomy.

Skeletal System

This is the basic structure of the body. It's composed of 206 bones, as well as the joints and cartilage that form them. There are general aspects we must understand about the skeletal system before we dive into the details, so first of all, we should know it looks like this:

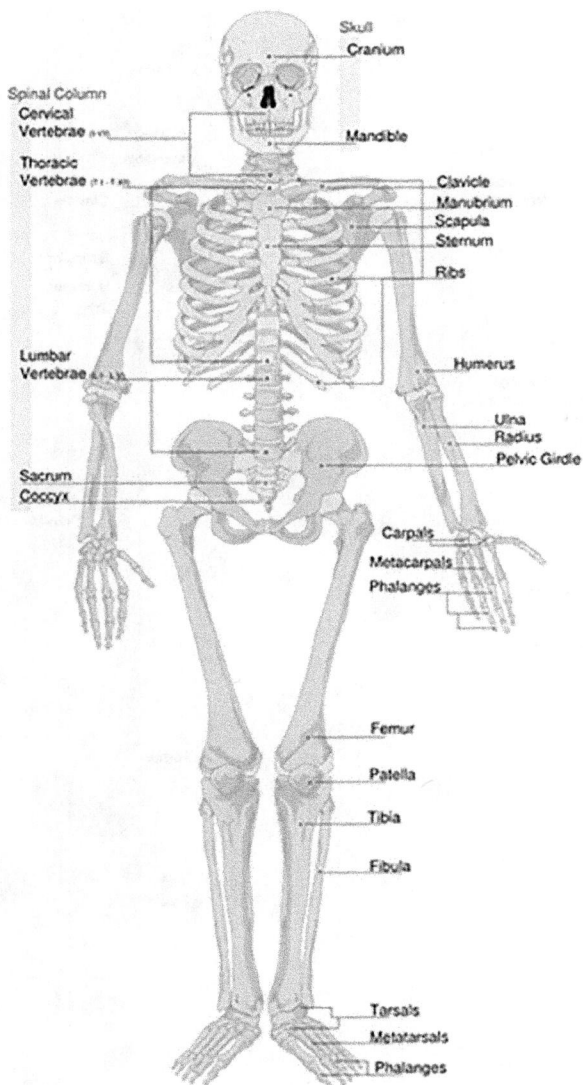

Skull
Cranium

Spinal Column
Cervical
Vertebrae (1-VII)

Mandible

Thoracic
Vertebrae (T1-T XII)

Clavicle
Manubrium
Scapula
Sternum
Ribs

Lumbar
Vertebrae (L-1-LV)

Humerus

Ulna
Radius
Pelvic Girdle

Sacrum
Coccyx

Carpals
Metacarpals
Phalanges

Femur
Patella
Tibia
Fibula

Tarsals
Metatarsals
Phalanges

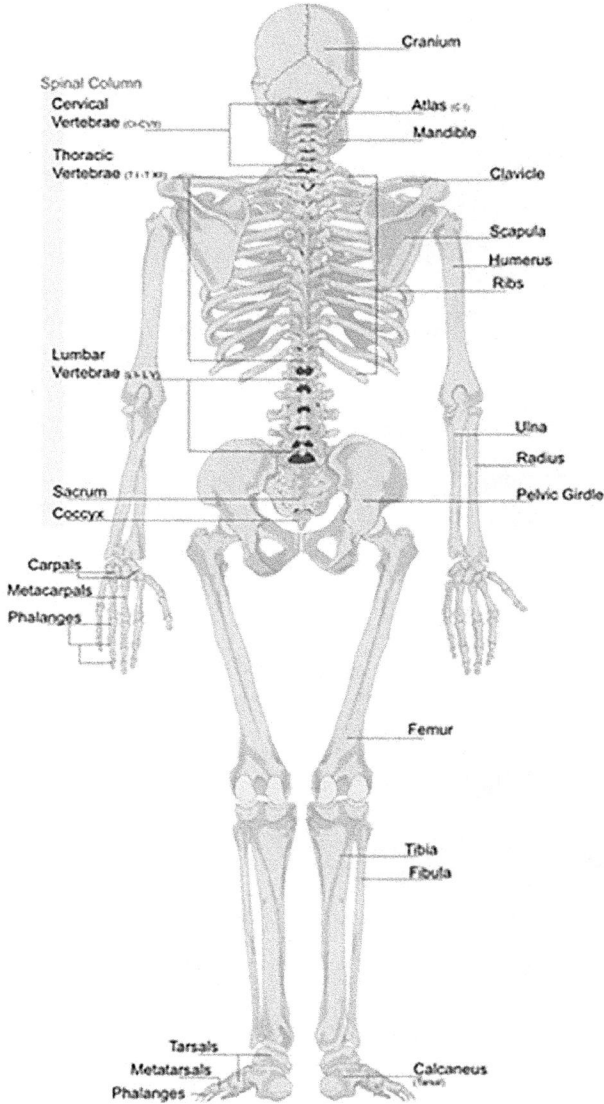

Cranium

Spinal Column
Cervical Vertebrae (C1-CV8)

Atlas (C-1)

Mandible

Thoracic Vertebrae (T1-T12)

Clavicle

Scapula

Humerus

Ribs

Lumbar Vertebrae (L1-LV5)

Ulna

Radius

Sacrum

Pelvic Girdle

Coccyx

Carpals

Metacarpals

Phalanges

Femur

Tibia

Fibula

Tarsals

Metatarsals

Calcaneus (Tarsal)

Phalanges

The basic way to divide the skeletal system is between the axial skeleton and the appendicular skeleton.

The axial skeleton is formed by the vertical axis of the skeletal system, which basically goes from the top of the skull to the bottom of the coccyx. It's composed of the skull, the vertebral column, and the ribcage.

The appendicular skeleton, unlike the previous one, is composed of the bones that hold the extremities, as well as those intended to attach the limbs to the axial skeleton. This means that the pelvis, scapula, and clavicle are all part of the appendicular skeleton.

This picture will illustrate the difference between the axial skeleton and the appendicular skeleton. We'll see the axial skeleton in white color, and the appendicular skeleton in red color.

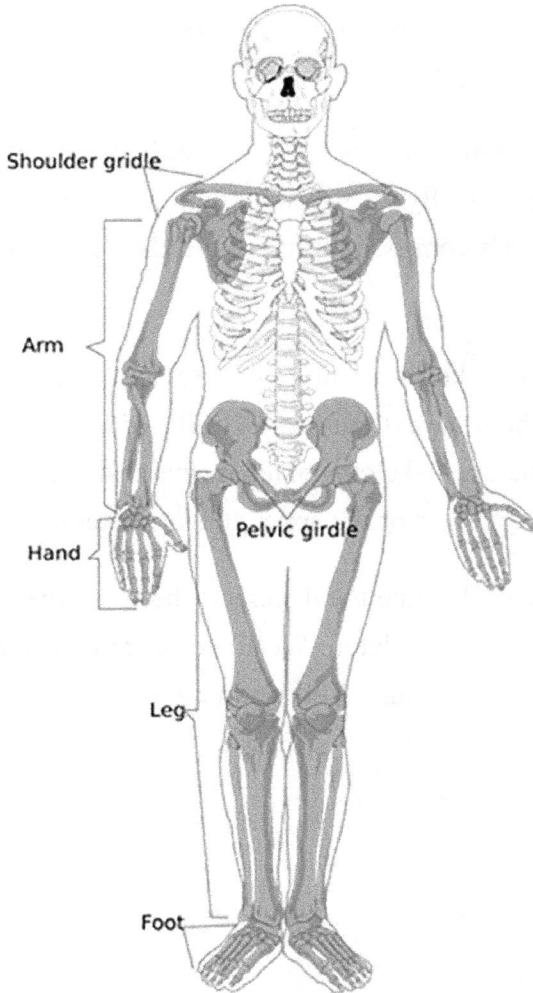

Axial Skeleton

The axial skeleton holds the body's most vital organs and structures, so it's important to understand where these structures are located and how the bones around them protect them. First of all, we have the skull:

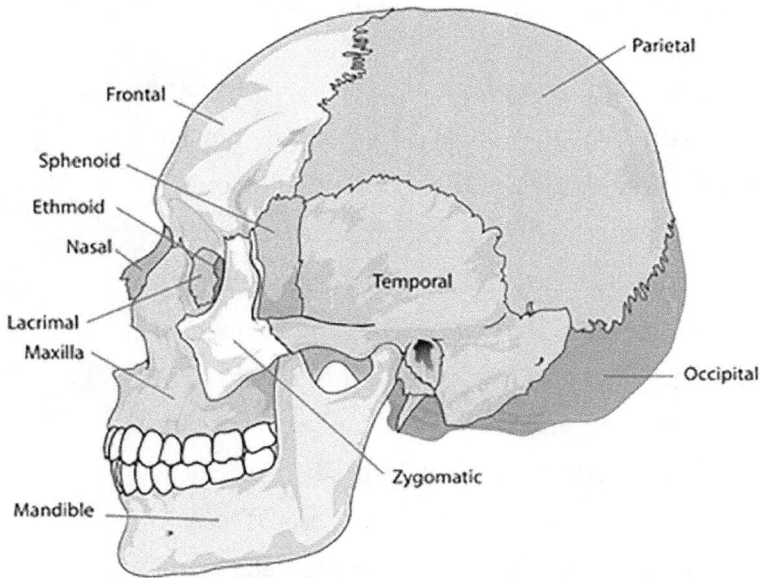

It holds the body's most important organ, the brain, inside of the neurocranium. What you need to know about the skull is that, even though the bones that form it are fairly strong to give our brain some extra protection, it still has some parts that are particularly weak and prone to fractures. The Zygomatic bones, the Temporal articulation with the Zygomatic bone (the horizontal part of the Temporal bone that goes out to meet the Zygomatic), and the Sphenoid bones are all prone to fracture. Also, the sutures of the skull, that is, the lines that join the different bones of the cranium, are weak spots. If you pay attention, there's a particularly weak area in the union between the Frontal, Parietal, Temporal, and Sphenoid bone, so any kind of traumatism that you see in that part of the skull must be investigated. Also, blunt force applied to the skull can still damage the structures inside if it's strong enough; this applies to the skull, as well as the eyeballs that lie inside of the orbital cavities.

Below the skull, we have the whole vertebral column. This is composed of 34 vertebrae, but the number can vary between 32 to 35 depending on the length of the coccyx. These vertebrae are different, and they grow sturdier and larger as they approach the bottom to make sure they're strong enough to sustain the weight of the body. This means that inferior vertebrae are stronger and more enduring than superior vertebrae. There are seven cervical vertebrae (neck), twelve thoracic vertebrae (thorax), five lumbar vertebrae (abdomen), five (fused) sacral vertebrae (pelvis), and four (fused) coccygeal vertebrae. There are intervertebral discs between each individual vertebrae. You may see a representation of the vertebral column in the next picture.

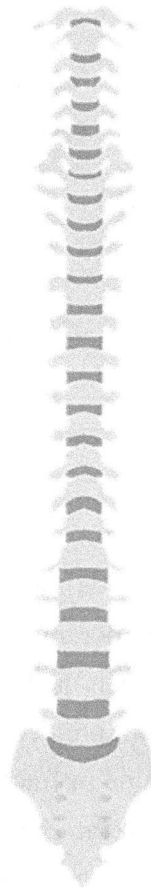

The most relevant aspect of the vertebral column is that it holds and protects the spinal cord. The spinal cord is the part of the central nervous in charge of connecting the peripheral nervous system to the encephalon. If any of the vertebrae is severely damaged, or an intervertebral disc, the spinal cord is injured. An injury of the spinal cord disconnects everything below the injury from the brain, which could leave the patient paralyzed if the damage is irreversible. Remember that the lower vertebrae are sturdier and stronger than the higher vertebrae, so the patient's neck is more vulnerable than the patient's pelvis. This knowledge is relevant to assess injuries and immobilize patients to transport them.

In the middle of the body, inferior to the neck, we have the thoracic cage. It's composed of the thoracic vertebrae in the posterior, twelve pairs of ribs at each side of the thorax, and the sternum forms the anterior wall, as you may see in the picture of the skeleton. The thorax is heavily guarded with bones to protect vulnerable structures inside of them. These structures are the lungs and the heart. Many people believe that the heart is placed on the left side of the chest, but that's not true. The heart is interior to the sternum because that's its function, to protect the heart from injuries. The ribcages are there to protect the lungs, vital organs that are also extremely vulnerable.

The relevance of this knowledge is to have an idea of the possibly affected organs behind a gunshot to the chest. As we'll see in the fourth chapter, those bullets of small caliber are capable of bouncing over hard structures, so a gunshot to the chest with a small entrance found, without an exit wound at the other side, may have bounced over one of the ribs. The bullet's trajectory and possible exit wound must be located to have an idea of the injured organs. Also, a fractured rib can pierce the lung, so that should also be considered when you evaluate patients.

Appendicular Skeleton

The body's extremities form this. The only vital structures that run around these bones are the main blood vessels, and these will be covered in a separate section. However, it's still important to learn the names of these bones to use them as an anatomical reference.

The scapulas are the bones commonly referred to as the "shoulder blades." These bones lie behind the thoracic cage, and its main function is to facilitate the movement of the arms. In front of the thoracic cage lie two long bones that go from the sternum to the shoulders. These are called clavicles, but you may know them by the name of "collar bones." These bones give stability to the arms. They're rather fragile and could be fractured in an accident, injuring essential arteries that run behind them, so we have to be careful with these bones during the patient's examination. The first bone of the arm, the humerus, goes from the shoulder articulation to the elbow, where it meets the radius (located laterally in the anatomical position) and ulna (located medially in the anatomical position). Then we have the carpal bones, metacarpal bones, and phalanges, which compose the hands.

There's a very similar structure in the legs. You have the pelvis, which is the large bone articulated with the sacrum. It supports our weight, protects our pelvic organs, and is articulated with the largest bone of the body, the femur. The femur is similar to the humerus, but it's much larger. You have the tibia and fibula distal from the femur, just like the radius and ulna in the forearm. The tibia is located medially, and the fibula is lateral to the tibia. Then you have the tarsal bones, metatarsal bones, and phalanges, which form the feet. It's important to highlight that bullets can bounce up from the femur and into the pelvis cavity, so an exit wound is important, even when we're dealing with wounds in the legs.

Nervous System

As we'll see in the next chapter, the nervous system is one of the systems in charge of controlling our body functions. It's extremely vulnerable, and we already know where it's located thanks to the bones that cover them. Still, we must understand some things regarding the nervous system to assess what's going on in the body of an injured patient.

The brain is the center of conscience, memory, and reason. The cerebral cortex, the most superficial part of the brain, has differentiated lobes dedicated to different functions of the body.

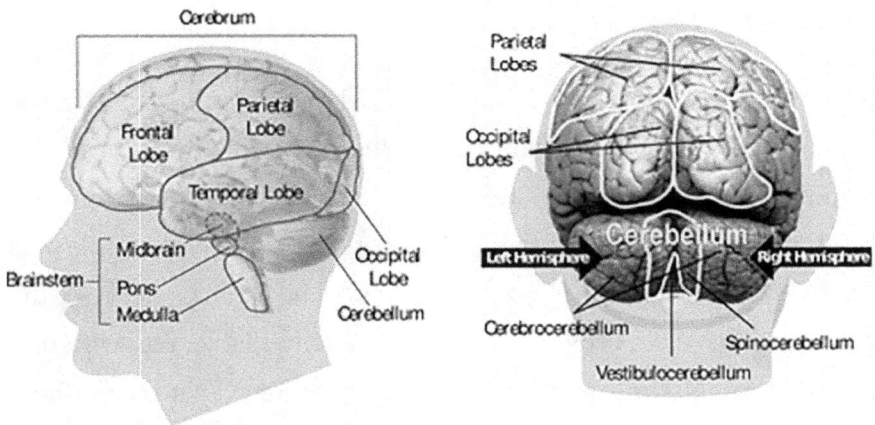

This is relevant because any injuries will manifest in the different symptoms presented by the patient. The frontal lobe is in charge of superior language and behavior, while the parietal lobe is in charge of movement. The temporal lobe is in charge of lower language functions such as understanding language, as well as hearing, and the occipital lobes are in charge of vision. So, for example, if a patient is injured in the back of the head and is currently unable to see, you should think about an occipital lobe injury.

There's another important concept that we have to understand, and it's the intracranial pressure. The central nervous system is surrounded by cerebrospinal fluid, which nurtures the nervous tissue and protects it by cushioning any hits. If there's bleeding due to an injury around the brain, the amount of fluid will rise, increasing the intracranial pressure. This will cause headaches, vomit, and sometimes even leakages of cerebrospinal fluid through the nose and ears. This is a very serious condition, and if it's not treated urgently, it can end the patient's life by pushing the brain towards the spine and harming the brainstem.

Running down the nervous system, we have the spinal cord. The spinal cord works as a data center that collects the information coming from the different parts of the body and sends the information from the encephalon to the body's organs. This information is transferred through the spinal nerves. The spinal nerves, the beginning of the peripheral nervous system, leave the vertebral column through the spaces between the vertebrae. This means there are five pairs of sacral nerves, five pairs of lumbar nerves, twelve pairs of thoracic nerves, eight pairs of cervical nerves, and, in the end, just one pair of coccygeal nerves. Each of these nerves is responsible for communication with a particular segment of the body. If the connection between a spinal nerve and the brain is severed, the person will no longer be able to feel that part of his body or move the muscles that were attached to that nerve. This may not be so relevant when the injury happens in the nerve; however, if the spinal cord is the one deeply affected, this will affect all of the spinal nerves inferior to the injury. If the spinal cord is severed, the patient won't be able to feel or move anything inferior to the injury. This is something we should always think about when we see traumatized patients that are unable to feel anything in a particular part of their bodies.

Circulatory System

The circulatory system is responsible for taking the blood around the body. Blood in the arteries is rich with oxygen and nutrients, and our body tissues are unable to survive without oxygen, especially the brain, so any failure in the circulatory system is a life-threatening situation. First of all, we should talk about the organ responsible for pumping blood through our bodies.

The Heart

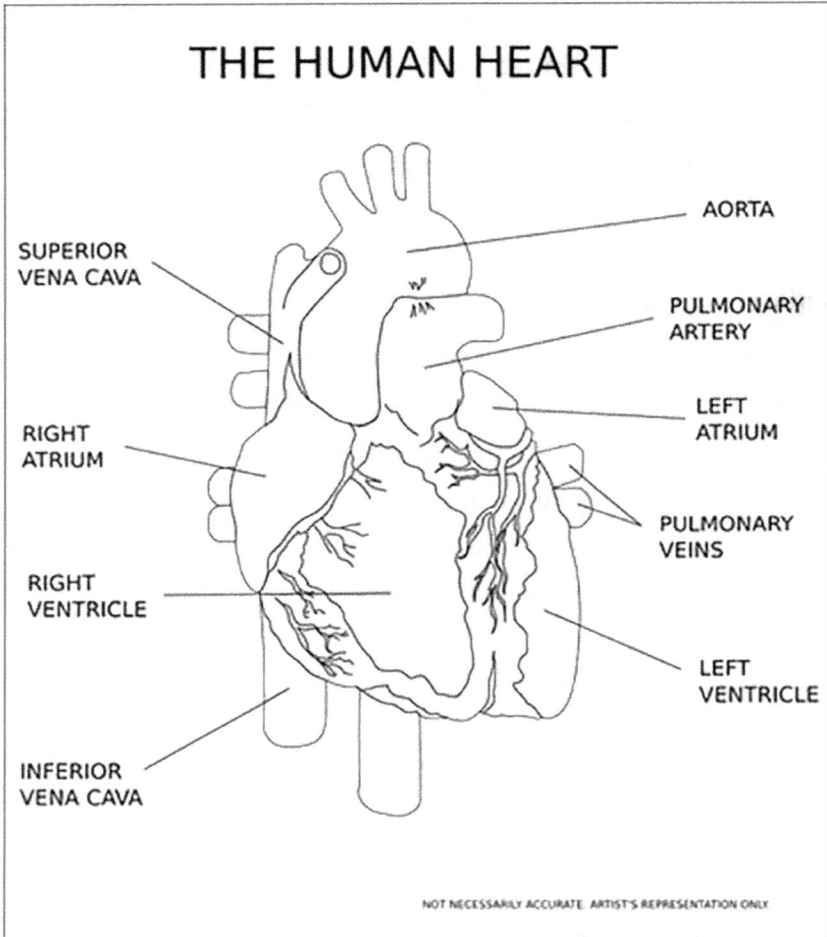

THE HUMAN HEART

SUPERIOR VENA CAVA

AORTA

PULMONARY ARTERY

LEFT ATRIUM

RIGHT ATRIUM

PULMONARY VEINS

RIGHT VENTRICLE

LEFT VENTRICLE

INFERIOR VENA CAVA

NOT NECESSARILY ACCURATE. ARTIST'S REPRESENTATION ONLY

The heart is the most important organ in the circulatory system. The right side of the heart receives the blood from the body in the right atrium; then it pushes it towards the lungs with the right ventricle. This venous blood is oxygenated in the lungs, and then it's received as arterial blood by the heart in the left atrium, passed over to the left ventricle, and pumped out towards the body through the aorta. This is the reason why people who receive a gunshot directly to the heart can't be saved. If the heart is severely ruptured, the patient will lose all of his body's blood through the rupture. Also, he'll be unable to pump blood towards his brain.

There's a bag of tissue covering the heart called the pericardium. This bag of tissue is formed of two walls; the inner wall is attached to the heart, and the outer wall is attached to everything around it (the lungs, sternum, thoracic spine, and other structures). These walls are usually attached to one another, but if the pericardium is injured, it can be filled with blood and other fluids, a syndrome known as pericardial effusion. If the amount of fluid inside the pericardium becomes too large, it can even compress the heart, suppressing its functions. This is a very dangerous situation because it causes severe hypotension. Other than that, it needs professional devices to be properly diagnosed and treated, so the paramedic can only have an idea of what's happening and take the patient to a specialized trauma center.

Arteries and Veins

As a general rule, arteries are the blood vessels that carry arterial blood towards the organs. Veins are the body's blood vessels responsible for recovering venous blood from the organs and taking it back to the heart. Arteries are born from the heart and run towards the peripherals of the body. Veins are born at the end of the arteries, and they return this blood to the heart.

Arterial blood is filled with oxygen, and it has a bright red color because that's the color of hemoglobin when it's carrying oxygen. It also flows with the heart pulses, causing arterial bleeding will shoot out of the injuries in rhythmic motions with every heartbeat. If the blood is bright red, and it's shooting out of the wound in short bursts, then you know that the affected blood vessel is an artery.

Venous blood, on the other hand, is filled with carbon dioxide. This blood takes a darker color, the color of hemoglobin that's not carrying oxygen. Unlike arterial blood, the venous blood doesn't shoot out in short bursts from wounds. This happens because the venous blood pressure doesn't rely as much on the heart. Instead, it relies on the muscles of the body to pump the blood back to the right atrium. This means that, if the blood is dark, and it's flowing steadily out of the wound, you know that the ruptured blood vessel is a vein.

Knowing whether the injured blood vessel is an artery or a vein will change the way to stop the bleeding, so it's important to be able to recognize arterial and venous blood when you see it.

Important Blood Vessels

The circulatory system is composed of veins and arteries are larger the closer they get to the heart, and smaller when they reach their final destinations (for the arteries) or start flowing from their starting points (when we talk about the veins). The bigger the blood vessel, the greater the blood loss, so it's important to know at least the location of the greatest blood vessels in the body.

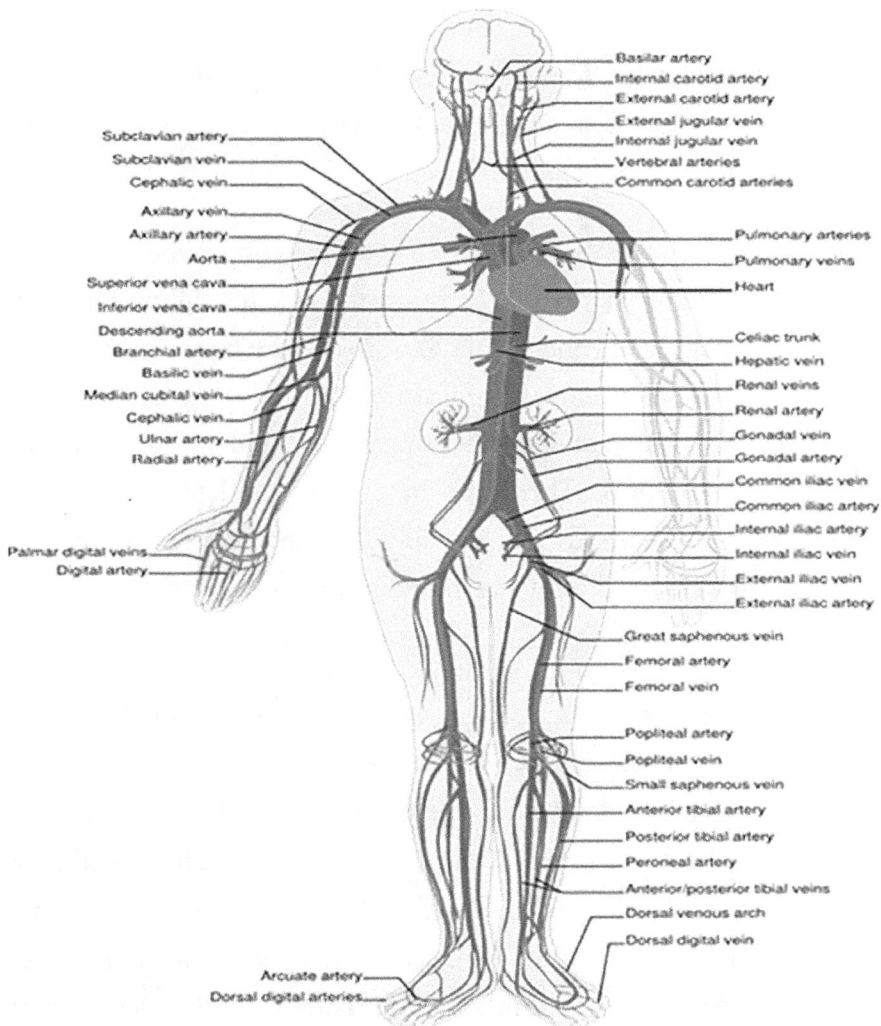

Basilar artery
Internal carotid artery
External carotid artery
External jugular vein
Internal jugular vein
Vertebral arteries
Common carotid arteries

Subclavian artery
Subclavian vein
Cephalic vein
Axillary vein
Axillary artery
Aorta
Superior vena cava
Inferior vena cava
Descending aorta
Branchial artery
Basilic vein
Median cubital vein
Cephalic vein
Ulnar artery
Radial artery

Palmar digital veins
Digital artery

Pulmonary arteries
Pulmonary veins
Heart

Celiac trunk
Hepatic vein
Renal veins
Renal artery
Gonadal vein
Gonadal artery
Common iliac vein
Common iliac artery
Internal iliac artery
Internal iliac vein
External iliac vein
External iliac artery

Great saphenous vein
Femoral artery
Femoral vein

Popliteal artery
Popliteal vein
Small saphenous vein
Anterior tibial artery
Posterior tibial artery
Peroneal artery
Anterior/posterior tibial veins
Dorsal venous arch
Dorsal digital vein

Arcuate artery
Dorsal digital arteries

The aorta is the body's main artery. It takes the arterial blood from the heart to the peripherals of the body. It's born right over the heart, posterior to the sternum, and then it goes slightly left and down in a straight line until it bifurcates at the limit between the fifth lumbar and the first sacral vertebrae. Both internal iliac arteries are born from this bifurcation. Any injury to the higher levels of the aorta will most likely end the patient's life. But if the aorta is injured during its trajectory through the abdomen, it's sometimes possible to save the patient if he receives treatment as fast as possible. The rest of the arteries of the body all come from the aorta.

The brachiocephalic trunk comes out of the top of the aorta and divides itself between the right carotid artery and the right subclavian artery. The left carotid and subclavian arteries are born directly from the aorta. The carotid arteries raise through the neck and into the head. They're located at both sides of the neck, and they carry a very important blood flow. These are the arteries used to evaluate the pulse rate at the neck. Arterial bleeding from the neck should always be assumed to come from the rupture of a carotid artery, so it must be acted upon quickly.

The subclavian arteries run slightly below and behind the clavicles, searching to be protected by these bones. This is the reason why a fractured clavicle should alert the clinicians of the possibility of internal bleeding. Both subclavian arteries follow this path until they cross the lateral border of the first rib. At this limit, they become the axillary arteries for a short distance until they're called brachial arteries. These run by the arm's surface, anterior to the biceps, then they cross over laterally until they reach the antecubital fossa. This last location is the one we use to measure blood pressure with a sphygmomanometer. When it reaches the elbow, it's divided between the radial artery (lateral) and the ulnar artery (medial). The radial arteries are the ones used to measure pulse rate in the forearms. It's important to remember the location of these blood vessels to assess injuries. We know that an injury anterior to the biceps is serious because it may rupture the brachial artery, for example.

The aorta doesn't give any relevant branches at the rest of its trajectory through the thoracic cavity. There are many relevant arteries in the abdominal trajectory of the aorta, such as renal arteries and mesenteric arteries. These carry a very important blood flow, but they're harder to locate, so there's not a high clinical value in understanding where they are. All you need to know is that penetrating wounds to the abdomen could harm these arteries, and it'll show with tachycardia and hypotension, so all patients with penetrating wounds to the abdomen are considered to be in critical conditions unless proven otherwise.

Then we have the common iliac arteries, these are the result of the bifurcation of the aorta, and they supply the pelvis legs with arterial blood. The internal iliac arteries supply the pelvis. These arteries are inferior to the pelvis and reproductive organs; the external iliac arteries are much more relevant to the body. They proceed inferior and anterior in a superficial trajectory until they exit the pelvis anterior to the pelvic tubercle, at which point they're called femoral arteries. Femoral arteries descend through an anteromedial trajectory to the thigh, so that's the most vulnerable part of the leg. Then they turn internally towards the popliteal fossa and become popliteal arteries. These also carry an important blood flow, but they're deeper than femoral arteries, so they're not as vulnerable to injuries.

This is as far as we must go studying the body's main arteries. The veins usually run next to the arteries; they're just deeper than them.

So if you know where to find the brachial artery, you'll probably know the location of the associated vein that runs with it. The differences appear in the larger veins. The counterpart of the aorta would be the cava veins. These collect the venous blood from the whole body and take it to the right atrium. They're deep in the body, and they follow a path similar to that of the aorta, only that the inferior cava vein runs upward to the heart, while the superior cava vein collects the blood from the head and gets it downwards to the heart.

This may seem like an overwhelming amount of information, but in some circumstances, it can be the difference between life and death. Also, it's impossible to apply a bandage and stop bleeding correctly if you're not sure about the ruptured blood vessel, so it's worth the effort to learn about the main arteries and veins of the human body.

Respiratory System

The respiratory system is the one responsible for taking oxygen and taking out carbon dioxide through our breathing. It's composed of the nose, nasal cavities, sinuses, pharynx, larynx, trachea, and lungs. The mouth is also considered to be part of the respiratory system, and other systems like the digestive system.

The respiratory system is key to our survival. If any of the organs involved are injured, the patient may die from asphyxia. It's impossible to restore the airways of a traumatized patient if you don't have a basic knowledge of the anatomy of some of the components of this system, so you should study it carefully.

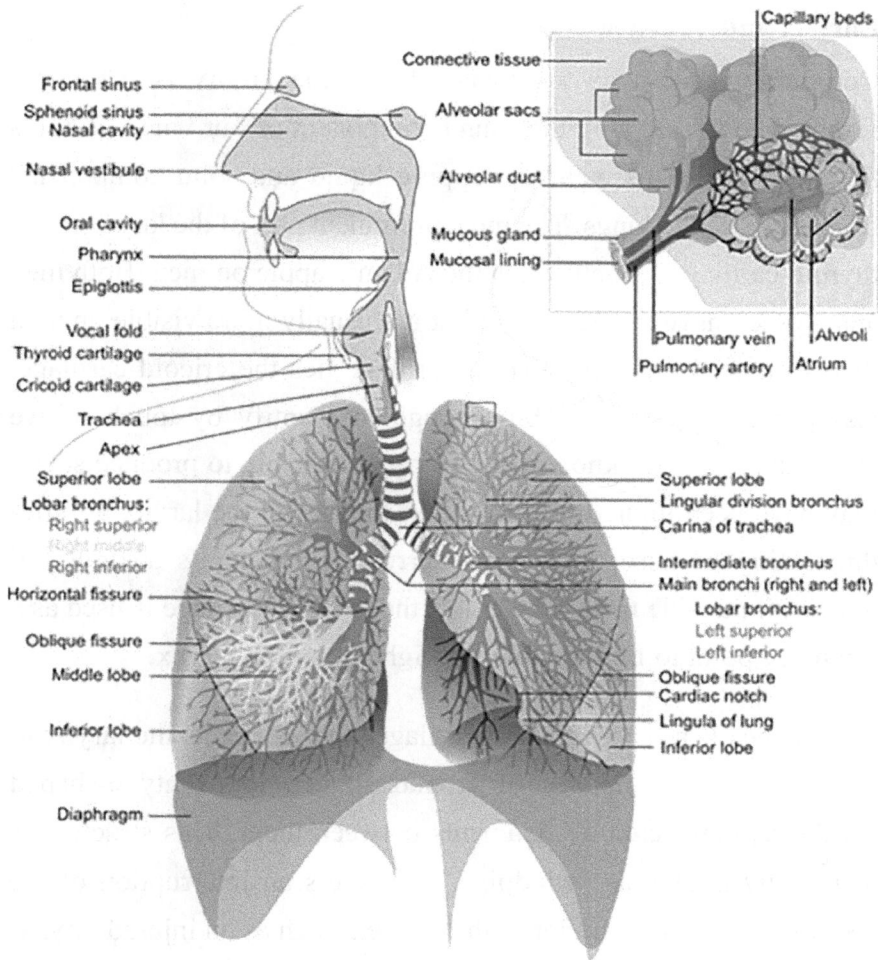

Frontal sinus
Sphenoid sinus
Nasal cavity
Nasal vestibule
Oral cavity
Pharynx
Epiglottis
Vocal fold
Thyroid cartilage
Cricoid cartilage
Trachea
Apex
Superior lobe
Lobar bronchus:
    Right superior
    Right middle
    Right inferior
Horizontal fissure
Oblique fissure
Middle lobe
Inferior lobe
Diaphragm

Connective tissue
Alveolar sacs
Alveolar duct
Mucous gland
Mucosal lining

Capillary beds
Pulmonary vein
Pulmonary artery
Alveoli
Atrium

Superior lobe
Lingular division bronchus
Carina of trachea
Intermediate bronchus
Main bronchi (right and left)
Lobar bronchus:
    Left superior
    Left inferior
Oblique fissure
Cardiac notch
Lingula of lung
Inferior lobe

Inferior to the oral cavity, you'll find the pharynx, commonly known as the throat. Just like the mouth, the pharynx is part of both the respiratory system and the digestive system. Both systems are separated by the larynx. After that, you have the trachea leading to the lungs, and the esophagus posterior to the trachea, leading to the stomach.

Larynx and Trachea

Commonly known as the "voice box," the larynx is the organ responsible for creating the sound component of our voice (it holds the vocal folds), as well as stopping liquid and solid components from entering the lungs. The most prominent part of the larynx is the thyroid cartilage, which forms the Adam's apple on men. Both men and women have this structure, but it's usually more visible on men than women. Under the thyroid cartilage lies the cricoid cartilage, less prominent, but also big enough to identify by touch. If we understand this, we know that any patient unable to produce sound may have been injured in the larynx. Injuries to the larynx are life-threatening because they may interrupt the patient's airflow and render him unable to breathe. Also, the thyroid cartilage is used as a reference point to find the trachea, right under the larynx.

The trachea is a tube made of cartilages that connects the larynx to the lungs. It's composed of around sixteen to twenty c-shaped cartilages, connected by ligaments between them. This structure is commonly known as "windpipe." If there's an interruption of the respiratory system superior to the trachea, such as an injured larynx, the patient will need a tracheotomy. This is an incision over the anterior wall of the trachea to place a tube that'll allow the patient to keep breathing. This procedure is typically practiced in a surgical room, and professionals perform it; however, in a life-or-death situation where there's no professional help available within miles, it's better to know how to do it than to let a traumatized patient die without trying.

Lungs and Pleura

These are the main respiratory organs of the body. The lungs are located at both sides of the heart, taking the majority of the thoracic cavity. Injured lungs can be filled with blood. However, there's a more common consequence of a piercing injury to these structures; pleural disorders such as hemothorax and pneumothorax.

The lungs, just like the heart, are covered by a bag formed by two walls of tissue. This structure that covers the lungs is called the pleura, and it enables the lungs to expand with the thorax and diaphragm as we inhale. The superficial wall of tissue or membrane is called the parietal pleura, and it's attached to the walls of the thoracic cavity. The deep wall of tissue or membrane is called visceral pleura, and it's attached to the lungs. Between the visceral pleura and the parietal pleura, there's a virtual space called the pleural sac or pleural cavity. It's virtual because both membranes are closely attached to each other until there's an injury that causes a separation between them. When the pleural cavity is injured, and it starts filling with air, that's called pneumothorax, and when it's filled with blood, that's a hemothorax. Either of these conditions could collapse the lungs and render the patient unable to breathe. These are life-threatening conditions, and they should be treated as soon as possible. You may imagine the pleura as the blue part of the following picture.

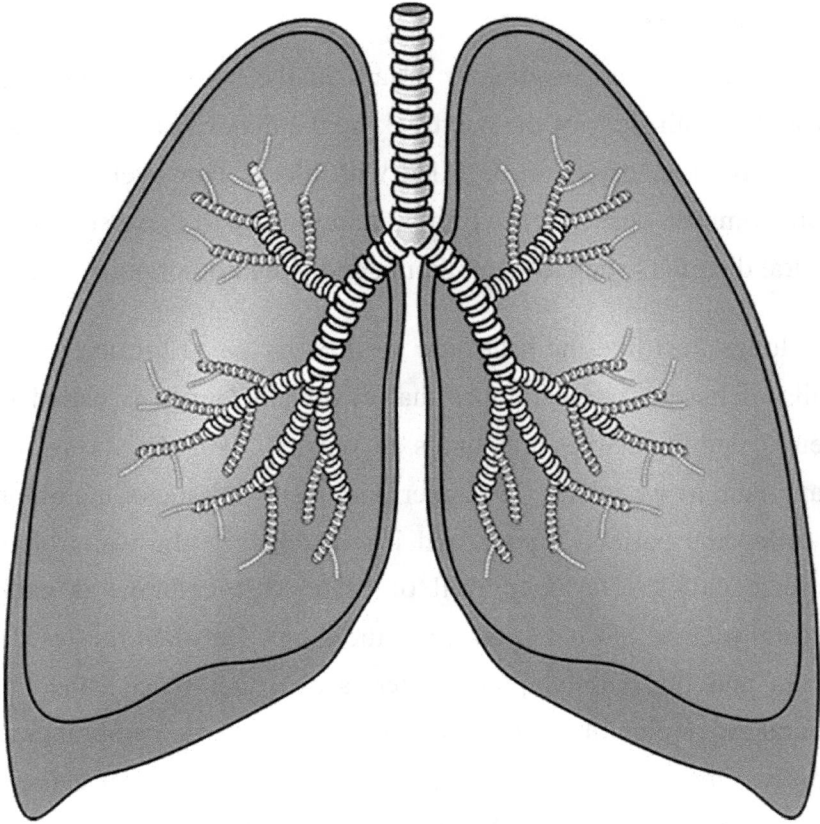

Abdominal Cavity

The rest of the systems of the body are less relevant in regard to gunshot wounds. The renal, digestive, and endocrine systems are only relevant for gunshot wounds to the abdominal cavity. So we're going to go through the vital organs that must be evaluated and addressed in traumatized patients, particularly the liver and the kidneys.

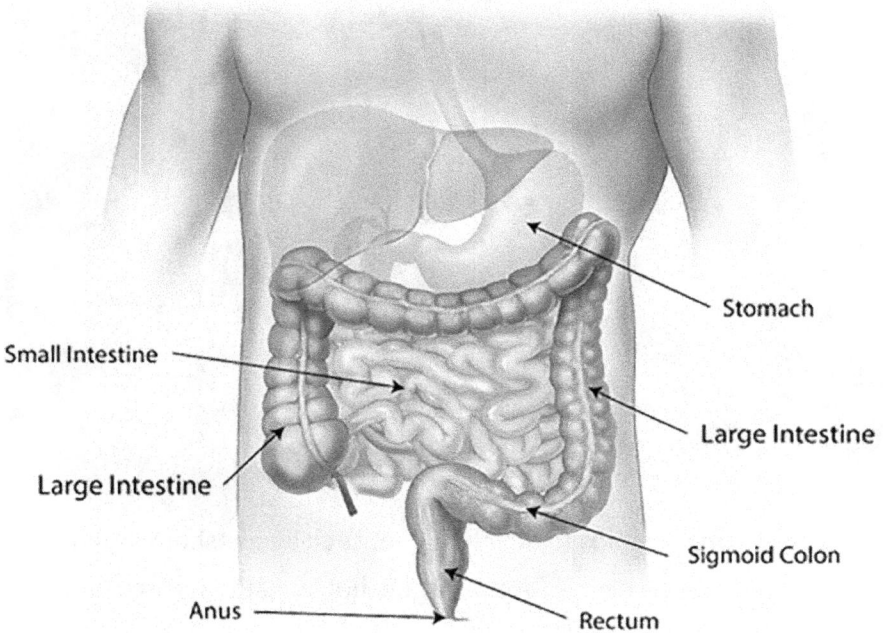

The liver, as you see in the image, is located at the top- right of the abdomen below the diaphragm. It works as the body's processing center. This means that most of our blood flow through the liver. A liver injury is a dangerous situation, and it must be addressed as fast as possible. These wounds can only be treated in a surgical room. The surgeons have to stop the bleeding and reconstruct the liver.

If the liver is an anterior structure that can be touched through the anterior abdominal wall, the kidneys are located to the posterior. They're inferior to your ribcage and irrigated by the renal arteries, which carry a great amount of blood.

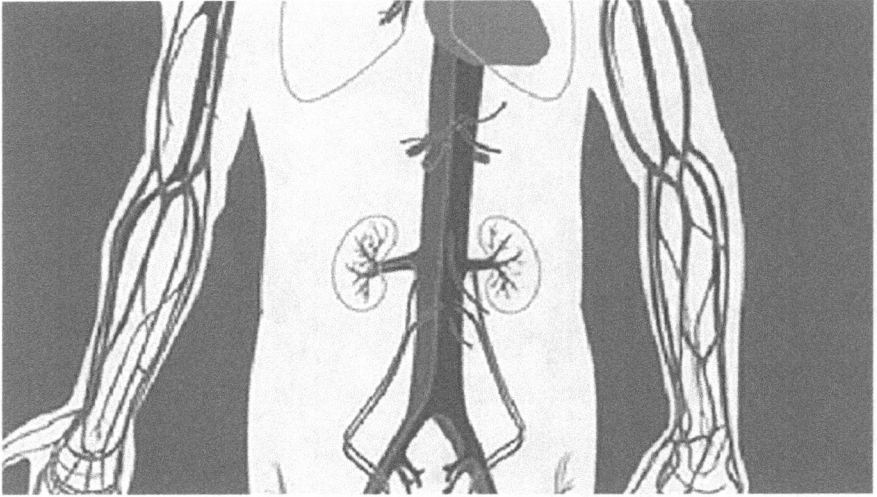

All penetrating wounds to the abdomen, such as gunshot wounds, are a reason to be alarmed. However, gunshot wounds located in these areas must be prioritized.

Applying the Knowledge

A great clinician who understands the anatomy always has a very good idea of what's going on with the traumatized patient at first sight. The location of the injury and the patient's symptoms and the condition is enough information to make a fast diagnosis and treat the damaged structure of the body, or at least limit the damage.

Chapter 3

The Unconscious Ruler
& Physiological Considerations

The human body is composed of extremely complex systems interacting with each other in harmony. Whenever one of the systems is damaged, the body responds to try to save the tissues and maintain balance. Clinicians study these responses as symptoms that tell us whether something's wrong or not and how to deal with the situation. Understanding how the body works are crucial to treating critical situations such as hypovolemic shock.

We have two systems responsible for controlling the rest of the body, the nervous system, and the endocrine system. Both send signals to the rest of the organs, telling them what to do and when to do it. The endocrine system is far slower than the nervous system. It still has its own value as a regulatory structure of the body, but its slow response speed makes it less relevant to manage critical injuries. Wound management is mainly the work of the nervous system, primarily the autonomic nervous system.

We can divide the nervous system as the central nervous system and peripheral nervous system anatomically, but there's a more relevant distinction functionally. The nervous system has a conscious and an unconscious component. If you move your hands, walk, talk, or perform any other conscious action, you're doing it from your somatic nervous system. This is your conscious component, the one that allows you to take action in your life. The autonomic nervous system, technically part of the peripheral nervous system, works by itself, just like any other system of your body. You can't control it any more than you can control your own stomach. It's important to understand the autonomic nervous system because there are many drugs used to treat traumatized patients that rely on this structure.

Depending on the sources you consult, you'll find that the autonomic nervous system is either divided between two or three branches. We have the sympathetic nervous system, parasympathetic nervous system, and enteric nervous system, or just the two former ones. The sympathetic nervous system is commonly known as the one responsible for the "fight or flight" reactions, while the parasympathetic nervous system works in a "feed and breed" situation. Their actions are opposite to one another because they're active in entirely opposite circumstances. We'll study the autonomic nervous system just as the sympathetic and parasympathetic nervous systems since both of these take charge of everything, particularly what's relevant for a traumatized patient.

Neurotransmitters

The nervous system communicates through chemical signals called neurotransmitters. These are chemical substances that are released by the nerves to transport information through the body, not unlike the energy and information flowing through your cables. Both the somatic and the autonomic nervous systems use neurotransmitters to communicate, but we're going to focus on the autonomic nervous system because of its relevance in the treatment of traumatized patients. The different neurotransmitters cause separated reactions to the body's tissues and organs. If the heart receives, for example, acetylcholine, it'll react completely differently than when it receives norepinephrine. The target organs of these chemical substances have specialized structures designed to receive them and interpret their signals. These structures are called receptors, and the diversification between them allows the body a wide array of actions and consequences from the stimuli of the nervous system. It's also important to point out that, since the autonomic nervous system is part of the peripheral nervous system, any neurotransmitters used by it won't have their usual consequences on the central nervous system. So, for example, acetylcholine released by the autonomic nervous system won't work as a neuromodulator because that's what it does in the central nervous system. This complex chemical code is used by the sympathetic and parasympathetic nervous systems as a way to communicate the information. The knowledge derived from studying these chemical substances and the receptors allows us to create drugs that'll either release or mimic the neurotransmitters, causing the effects we desire in the human body. There are two main neurotransmitters used by the autonomic nervous system. These are acetylcholine and norepinephrine.

Acetylcholine

The parasympathetic nervous system primarily uses this neurotransmitter. It works on the muscular tissue and the secretion of glands such as the digestive glands. It has different actions depending on the target organ and receptors it acts upon. It works on the nicotinic and muscarinic receptors.

Norepinephrine

Norepinephrine, commonly known as noradrenaline, is the main neurotransmitter of the sympathetic nervous system. It usually prepares our body for intense physical activity. Just like with acetylcholine, norepinephrine changes its functions depending on the target organs and receptors. It works on the alpha-1, alpha-2, and beta-1 receptors.

Epinephrine

It's the result of the methylation of norepinephrine to make epinephrine. It's technically not a neurotransmitter but a hormone because neurons do not transport them. However, they're released by the sympathetic nervous system, and they act on the sympathetic receptors, so they're still considered part of the autonomic nervous system. Commonly known as adrenaline, it's only secreted by the adrenal medulla of the suprarenal glands. It works similarly to norepinephrine, but it also affects beta-2 receptors.

Preganglionic and Postganglionic

Neural connections are made with a large web of intertwined neurons. The connection between these neurons is called a synapse. The way that the information runs through the nervous system is by a release of the neurotransmitters mentioned above. The releasing neuron is called presynaptic, while the receiving neuron is the postsynaptic neuron. When we speak about the autonomic nervous system, we have a vital structure called the autonomic ganglia. This is the place where the synapse between the central nervous system's neuron and the peripheral nervous system's neuron happens. Neurons located proximal to the ganglia are preganglionic and are the presynaptic neuron of that connection. They run down from the encephalon and the spinal cord until they reach the autonomic ganglia, located at both sides of the spinal cord. Neurons located distal to the ganglia are postganglionic and are the postsynaptic neurons in that connection. They receive the information from the autonomic ganglia and take it to the target organ. It's important to understand this because some neurotransmitters and hormones work differently depending on whether they're acting over a preganglionic or postganglionic neuron.

In a Time of Leisure

The sympathetic nervous system is in charge of our time of rest and peace. It's responsible for our "rest and digest" or "feed and breed" actions. We need it to process food, rest, sleep, and keep the body relaxed when we don't need to get moving. It's easier to understand what this system does if we divide it by its different actions.

Digestion

This is the main function of the parasympathetic nervous system. It enables peristalsis by activating the muscular fibers of the digestive tube. These are the movements performed by the digestive system to keep the digested food flowing towards the rectum. This transport is part of the digestive process. Without it, we wouldn't be able to absorb the nutrients from our food. The parasympathetic nervous system also activates the secretion of acid in the stomach, vital to transform and seize the nutrients present in our meals. Other glands related to the digestive system are activated by the parasympathetic, such as the pancreas. The relaxation of the sphincters is also activated by the parasympathetic nervous system, enabling the process of excretion.

Urination

The parasympathetic system contracts the muscles of the bladder and relaxes the sphincters, enabling the release of urine from the bladder.

Pupillary Response

The parasympathetic nervous system contracts the iris sphincter muscle, decreasing the size of the pupils. This adaptation is useful to avoid light to enter the eyes in environments filled by it. They also adapt the eyes for seeing close things.

Sexual Activity

The vasodilation of the arteries that flow towards the sexual organs prepares the human body for sexual intercourse. The parasympathetic nervous system controls this.

Respiration

The parasympathetic nervous system inhibits breathing. It contracts the muscles present in the airways, closing the channels used to transport air through the lungs. It also stimulates the secretion of mucus that'll block the passage of air. Hard breathing is not as necessary when the human body is relaxed.

Heart Activity

Heart rate is decreased, and blood pressure is lowered by the effect of the parasympathetic nervous system. It decreases the number of heart beats per minute, and it relaxes the heart's muscular tissue, making it weaker. There's no need to spend energy on an increased blood flow when the body's relaxed.

In a Time for Action

The sympathetic nervous system goes in an opposite direction than the parasympathetic nervous system. It's there to prepare us for action, which is the "fight or flight" reaction. Any human being under mental or physical stress will activate the sympathetic nervous system. This could be either from an injury, internal crisis, physical activity, or just plain excitement. The functions of the sympathetic nervous system will vary according to the target organ and tissue, but they'll all be directed in the same way.

Pupillary Response

The sympathetic nervous system acts upon the iris dilator muscle, making it contract. Instead of contracting the pupils, it dilates them, causing mydriasis. This way, the pupils grow bigger, taking more light from their environment and adapting to darker situations. It also adapts to seeing things that are far, which is traditionally more necessary for intense physical activity, especially primal survival activities such as hunting.

Breathing

The sympathetic nervous system relaxes the muscles around the airways, causing bronchodilation and enabling us to breathe better. Oxygen supply is extremely important for intense physical activity.

Heart Activity

The heart needs to beat faster and stronger in order to bring more blood to the tissues, particularly muscle tissue. The sympathetic nervous system increases the strength of the heart's muscle and the heart rate to enable the tissues to get more blood.

Blood Vessels

Blood not only needs to get faster towards its targets, but it also needs to be distributed differently. Physical activity demands blood in the muscular tissue, specifically skeletal muscle tissue, which is the one responsible for our movement. To get this effect, the sympathetic nervous system contracts the blood vessels on the skin, and abdominal organs such as the stomach and the intestine, and the kidneys. This reduces their blood supply and makes the blood travel faster through these blood vessels towards other destinations. Blood vessels located in skeletal muscle are, on the contrary, dilated by the action of the sympathetic nervous system. This allows this muscular tissue to receive more blood, and therefore, more oxygen.

Digestion

The sympathetic nervous system has an opposite effect over the digestive system than the parasympathetic nervous system. It inhibits peristalsis and gland secretion instead of enabling it. The energy of our bodies can't be wasted on digestion during physical activities. This is the reason why people shouldn't do any workouts right after eating.

Sweat Glands

Sweat can get confusing when we study the autonomic nervous system. Most gland secretion is enabled by the parasympathetic nervous system and inhibited by the sympathetic nervous system, except for sweat glands. The reason for this is that the sympathetic nervous system uses acetylcholine to activate these glands. The body has to avoid overheating during intense physical activity, so it uses sweat to cool down. The parasympathetic nervous system, as the main user of acetylcholine, is also capable of activating sweat glands. However, this is uncommon, for the connections between the nervous system and the sweat glands are mainly through the sympathetic nervous system unless there's something wrong.

Receptors

These are the specialized structures that receive the neurotransmitters and interpret their signals. Receptors can be found either on the cellular walls or inside of the cells, where they receive and process neurotransmitters. They can be divided between adrenergic and cholinergic receptors depending on the neurotransmitter used to activate them. However, some receptors can be activated by both kinds of neurotransmitters, provoking different effects on the human body.

Adrenergic Receptors

The adrenergic receptors are the alpha-1, alpha-2, beta-1, and beta-2 receptors. Alpha receptors are more abundant than beta receptors.

The alpha-1 receptors are excitatory, which means they enable a specific action (such as muscle contraction) on the target tissue. They're widely spread through the tissues of the body. They're activating receptors, so they tend to cause secretion and muscular contraction. They cause mydriasis and contract arterioles (with the exception of skeletal muscle's arterioles), among other functions.

Alpha-2 receptors, contrary to the alpha-1, are inhibitors. They work by avoiding an action, so they'll release muscular tension and relax the muscles, for example. They are distributed through the target tissues as well as the presynaptic neurons. It works by inhibiting its own release in the presynaptic neurons. This way, the sympathetic nervous system can be self-regulated.

All of the beta receptors can be either activators or inhibitors depending on their target tissue, just like muscarinic receptors. These are the primary adrenergic receptors of the heart (although some beta-2 receptors are working there as well). Both beta-1 and beta-2 receptors have an enabling activity in the heart, increasing its overall activity. They're equally activated by epinephrine and norepinephrine. Beta-1 receptors also enable the secretion of renin, which is a hormone that increases blood pressure.

Beta-2 receptors are the most common beta receptors in the target tissues. They can be activators or inhibitors, but they tend to be inhibitors. They're also more responsive to epinephrine than norepinephrine.

Cholinergic Receptors

These are the nicotinic and muscarinic receptors.

The nicotinic receptors are found on the postganglionic neurons of both the sympathetic and parasympathetic nervous systems. It activates these neurons, enabling them to carry their information towards their target organs and provoke a response.

The muscarinic receptors are found on the target tissues and organs. They're either activators or inhibitors depending on the tissue in which they're located. So, they'll activate the contraction of the airway muscular tissue, causing bronchoconstriction and thus, making breathing more difficult. However, they'll inhibit muscular contraction in the heart, decreasing its strength and, therefore, systolic blood pressure. There are five types of muscarinic receptors, called M-1, M-2, M-3, M-4, and M-5, respectively.

M-1 receptors work in the salivary glands, enabling the secretion of saliva. They also work on the stomach activating the release of stomach acid, helping the digestion. It's an activator.

M-2 receptors reduce heart rate and force of contraction. They're found in the heart tissue. This type of receptor is an inhibitor.

M-3 receptors are activators. They work on the muscular tissue of the lungs, provoking bronchoconstriction. They also provoke glandular secretion, such as salivation and stomach acid. They increase intestinal motility and peristalsis. They also contract the iris sphincter muscle, provoking miosis.

M-4 and M-5 aren't so important to the autonomic nervous system. M-4 receptors facilitate locomotion, which are the general movements of the body. M-5 receptors are only found in the central nervous system.

Table of Functions

It may be hard to keep track of all the different functions of the sympathetic and parasympathetic nervous systems, their neurotransmitters, the receptors, and the actions they perform over each one of these receptors. Here's a table to help you remember each one of these aspects.

Tissue	Receptor	Sympathetic Activity	Parasympathetic Activity
Iris sphincter muscle	M-3	No activity	Miosis

Iris dilator muscle	Alpha-1	Mydriasis	No activity
Ciliary muscle	Beta-2/M-3	Relaxation for far vision	Contraction for near vision
Heart	Beta-1, Beta-2 & Nicotinic /M-2	Increases heart rate Increases strength of the heart's muscle	Decreases heart rate Decreases strength of the heart's muscle
Skin arterioles	Alpha-1	Strong contraction	No activity
Abdominal arterioles	Alpha-1	Strong contraction	No activity
Kidney arterioles	Alpha-1	Strong contraction	No activity
Skeletal muscle arterioles	Alpha-1 & Beta-2	Mild contraction	No activity
Lungs airways	Beta-2/M-3	Bronchodilation	Bronchocon striction

Lungs glands	Alpha 1 & Beta-2/M-3	Decreases secretion of mucus	Increases secretion of mucus
Sweat glands	Muscarinic (1-5)	Generalized sweating	No activity under normal circumstances
Sweat glands	Alpha 1	Localized sweating	No activity
Adrenal medullae	Nicotinic	Increased secretion of epinephrine and norepinephrine	No activity
Salivary glands	Alpha-1 & Beta-2/M-3	Mild secretion of saliva	High secretion of saliva
Stomach motility	Alpha-1 & Beta-2/M-3	Decreased	Increased
Stomach secretion of acid	M-1 & M-3	No activity	Stimulation
Stomach sphincters	Alpha-1/M-3	Contraction	Relaxation

Intestine motility	Alpha-1 & Beta-2/M-3	Decreased	Increased
Intestine secretion	M-1 & M-3	No activity	Stimulation
Intestine sphincters	Alpha-1/M-3	Contraction	Relaxation
Bladder wall	Beta-2/M-3	Relaxation	Contraction
Bladder sphincter	Beta-2/M-3	Contraction	Relaxation
Kidney	Beta-1	Renin secretion	No activity

The Body's System of Alarm

The autonomic nervous system works together with several sensors located in the body to keep track of the body's condition and react accordingly if anything's wrong. The endocrine system takes part in this regulatory system, answering to any dire circumstances as an attempt for life-preservation.

There's a structure located in the carotid sinuses called a baroreceptor. The baroreceptors are sensors that detect low blood pressure. If the body's blood pressure starts to decrease, they'll activate the sympathetic nervous system to deal with this issue as soon as possible. If, on the contrary, blood pressure starts to rise, baroreceptors will send an alarm signal so that the body can react using the parasympathetic (along with other systems).

If we go up towards the encephalon, we'll fin oxygen-chemo sensitive sites in the brainstem. These chemo sensitive structures work as sensors to detect low oxygen saturation in the blood. Once they detect this, they're wired to react as fast as possible by activating the sympathetic nervous system and securing a good supply of oxygen.

Also, a critical situation will turn up the alarms of anyone aware of what's going on. Living a dangerous situation will instantly activate the sympathetic nervous system, immediately securing a good supply of blood to the brain, as well as the skeletal muscles. This will be the case in any conscious patients with a gunshot wound. However, mental stress isn't needed to activate the sympathetic nervous system. An unconscious patient will still benefit from the resources of the sympathetic nervous system thanks to these natural sensors, as well as other natural signs of alarm, such as physical pain.

Heart Rate and Arrhythmia

The human heart is capable of beating on its own. If separated from the body, it'll continue beating until it starts failing and stops. This is thanks to small masses of specialized tissue capable of generating electrical currents on their own and stimulating the contraction of the heart's muscles. These small masses are called heart nodes. There are four different heart nodes, and each one of them is capable of producing their own rhythmic stimuli by themselves. Each of these nodes has its own rate of electrical stimuli per minute; since they're all connected, the fastest one usually takes charge of producing heartbeats by carrying his electrical stimuli towards the others. These nodes are:

- The sinoatrial node, located at the top of the right atrium and connected to the atrioventricular node

- The atrioventricular node, located between the atriums and connected with the sinoatrial node

- The atrioventricular bundle, located between the two ventricles and connected with the atrioventricular node

- The purkinje fibers, located at the external walls of the ventricles and connected with the atrioventricular bundle.

The sinoatrial node is referred to as the heart's pacemaker because it's usually in charge of the heart's contractions. It has a stimuli rate of around 60 to 100 stimuli per minute, having the highest rate per minute. This node carries the electrical stimuli towards the subsequent nodes, causing the contraction of the heart muscles, and thus, a heartbeat. These stimuli are usually regular and symmetrical. The nodes don't pulse erratically; instead, the heartbeats are rhythmic and symmetrical because the nodes work that same way. The autonomic nervous system accelerates and decelerates heartbeats by directly influencing the activity of these nodes.

This is the way the electrical component of the heart works under normal circumstances. However, there are certain conditions, such as heart injury and the use of drugs that could alter the work of the nodes. When the sinoatrial node is unable to generate effective pulses, the next node takes over the heart's activity. That means that the atrioventricular node takes over the direction of the heartbeats; if it fails, the atrioventricular bundle takes over, and so on. Since each of these nodes has a slower rate than the previous one, the heart starts beating slower, causing bradycardia. Also, whenever a node stops pulsing rhythmically, the heart starts beating erratically (or, in serious cases, not beating at all). Both tachycardia, bradycardia, and irregular heartbeats fall into the definition of arrhythmia, and it's a serious condition that needs to be addressed and treated by specialized physicians. An arrhythmia where the stimuli are ruled by either the sinoatrial or atrioventricular nodes is called a supraventricular arrhythmia, and if it's ruled by either the atrioventricular bundle of the Purkinje fibers, it's ventricular arrhythmia.

There's another relevant condition in which none of the nodes will be creating electrical stimuli. The heart will lack electrical activity, and therefore, there won't be any heartbeats. This is called asystole, and it's a life-threatening situation that'll take the patient's life if not treated immediately.

Arrhythmias and asystole can't be identified without an electrocardiogram (or EKG). Electrocardiograms are tests that measure the electrical activity in the heart. If the nodes are still working, the EKG will detect and measure their activity even if the heart's no longer beating. An electrocardiogram is needed to identify whether arrhythmia is supraventricular or ventricular and if it's a tachyarrhythmia (tachycardia) or bradyarrhythmia (bradycardia).

The relevance of this knowledge is that some drugs can't be supplied to someone suffering from arrhythmia. Drugs such as atropine make some arrhythmias worse, so they can't be administered to a person with this sort of condition. This is the reason why administering drugs is such a delicate matter, and it's restricted to physicians.

Using this Knowledge

Physicians need to understand the autonomic nervous system, neurotransmitters, receptors, and their functions in order to treat a wide range of conditions. However, this knowledge is also vital for paramedics and other critical health professionals who need to practice cardiopulmonary resuscitation. As we'll learn in chapter six, there are drugs used by professionals during the process of cardiopulmonary resuscitation. These drugs either activate the sympathetic nervous system or inhibit the parasympathetic nervous system, so it's important to understand what these systems do before any attempt to use them. The use of these drugs is legally reserved for physicians and health professionals in most countries. However, in a life-or-death situation where there's no other resource available than to use one of these drugs; knowing how to administer them can save a life.

Chapter 4

Gunshot Wounds

Not all firearms use the same bullets or cause the same damage. Bullets usually provoke piercing wounds, but the consequences of these wounds may be very different according to the place of impact, the proximity, the kind of firearm, and the kind of bullet. A trained paramedic knows how to identify a gunshot wound in a matter of seconds, priceless information that must be gathered before attempting to heal the gunshot wound and save a life.

Penetrating and Perforating Wounds

Penetrating gunshot wounds are wounds with an entrance point, but no exit point. Perforating gunshot wounds, on the other hand, have both entrance and exit wounds. In the case of penetrating gunshot wounds, it's necessary to extract the bullet or bullet fragments from the patient's body in order to treat it. This can be very difficult, especially without adequate equipment and surgical training. Also, whenever you're dealing with a gunshot injury, if you can't see the entrance and exit wounds, you can't be sure about the bullet's trajectory. If the bullet hits bone, it can ricochet and change direction. Perforating gunshot wounds, on the other hand, never have this problem. However, the larger trajectory through the body increases the risk of damaged tissue.

Identifying the Distance

The distance between the gun's muzzle (the end of the barrel of the gun) and the injured person changes the damage and possible outcome. Closer distances will enter the body with more strength. This means that the organs and structures around the bullet's trajectory are more likely to be damaged the closer the distance between the wound and the muzzle; this is especially true around the entry wound. On the other hand, entering with more force through the body will make it less likely for the bullet to bounce off if it meets resistance. So, if a bullet finds a bone in its trajectory, it's more likely to break it and stay on course than to bounce off in a different direction if the muzzle was close to the injured person. Neither of these circumstances is positive for the patient's outcome, but the chance of bouncing off isn't too high, while the damage of a bullet shot at close range is always a reason to worry. This means that patients with a long-distance gunshot wound have a better chance at recovery. Identifying these injuries is done by examining the entrance wound.

Contact

Contact gunshot wounds are those in which the attacker sank the muzzle of the gun in the patient's flesh before he pulled the trigger. There are two possible ways in which these wounds can be identified.

If the contact wound happened in any place other than the skull, the wound will be perfectly round and have a seared and blackened skin margin. This blackened and seared margin happens because of the contact of the skin with the powder and the explosion.

A contact gunshot wound to the skull will behave differently because the skin is stretched out, covering the skull tightly. There are three different ways in which these wounds could appear. The wound could be just like the previous one, round with seared blackened margins. It can be a starred shape, which happens when the expanding gas of the gunshot dissects and tears the skin. The third way in which it can appear is as a round wound with a muzzle imprint; this is a gunshot wound that looks like the exit hole of the gun's barrel. In this last situation, the skin is pressed back against the gun due to the expansion of gas.

Near Contact

These are gunshot wounds that happen in very similar circumstances as the contact gunshot wounds, but the muzzle isn't touching the skin of the patient. The muzzle, in this case, is less than one centimeter away from the patient's skin, so the firearm is still held close enough to cause very similar internal damage as the contact wound. Near contact, wounds are identified as circular wounds with seared and blackened edges on the skin, only wider than the contact wounds.

Intermediate

The intermediate or close-range wounds are those close enough to leave a dark "powder tattoo" around the entrance wound. These gunshot wounds happen close enough that the powder leaving the gun's barrel is close enough to reach the skin. Depending on the firearm, these wounds can be caused by a distance of inches, up to a few feet. These wounds are identified because they don't cause laceration or muzzle imprint, but primarily because of the dark "powder tattoo" or powder stippling. It's important to point out that this powder stippling area is not a burned area. It's just covered with powder.

Distant

Distant wounds are far enough from the patient's skin that they don't leave a powder stippling. These are round gunshot wounds with an abrasion ring and sharp margins. The abrasion ring, unlike the contact wound, is not blackened. Also, there's no muzzle print or laceration. A distant gunshot wound also has a tendency to be smaller, being only as wide as the bullet.

The Trajectory of the Bullet

Most of the damage caused by a gunshot wound happens during the bullet's trajectory. The higher the deformation of the human body, the more damage caused by the bullet. Also, the more kinetic energy is carried by the bullet, the stronger the deformation, so we can say that kinetic energy is a defining factor in the bullet's damage. We've already talked about the bullet's proximity to the patient as a factor that alters the deformation caused by the bullet. Now we'll speak about two other relevant aspects: the speed and the shape of the bullet.

Speed of the Bullet

This is where the kind of weapon comes into the equation. All bullets are fast, but the gunshot of a handgun is much slower than that of an assault rifle. More speed means more kinetic energy, so a bullet fired by an assault rifle makes more damage than a bullet fired by a handgun, for example.

The Shape of the Bullet

There's a difference in the capacity of deformation between a hollow-point bullet, a flat bullet, and a full metal jacket bullet. Full metal jacket bullets don't have as much capacity for deformation as the other two. Instead, they're designed to slip easily through the body, provoke a perforating wound, and ricochet easily. Hollow-point bullets, on the other hand, have a high capacity of deformation, but they don't travel as much. So these bullets don't have a long trajectory; however, they usually do more damage in their limited area of effect. Flat bullets lie between hollow-point bullets and full metal jacket bullets.

Exit Wounds

Identifying exit wounds and telling them apart from entrance wounds isn't hard; there are a couple of qualities that are generally applied to exit wounds.

- The bullet finds it harder to burst out of the patient's body than it was to pierce in through the skin. This is because it may stumble during its trajectory through the patient's body, also, because it may become deformed due to an impact. This will be reflected in an exit wound more irregular than the entrance wound.

- The fragmentation of the bullet may divide it into smaller projectiles, creating smaller exit wounds around the main exit wound.

- Exit wounds don't have muzzle imprints, blackening of the edges of the skin, or powder stippling.

- Sometimes the patient has a "shored" exit wound. This happens when the bullet impacts something just as it leaves the patient's body; the skin was touching something else as the bullet pierced through it. Shored exit wounds are usually caused by hard materials such as walls. These exit wounds can be similar to distant entrance wounds because they also have an abrasion area. However, they'll be more irregular than the entrance wound, much smaller than a close-range entrance wound, and it won't have powder stippling.

Special Cases

Two particular situations don't usually fit with the rest of the gunshot injuries.

Keyhole Wounds

These are gunshot wounds where the entrance wound is the same as the exit wound. This can only happen when the bullet hits the skull at a shallow angle. The bullet never really enters the cranium, so it doesn't reach the brain. However, the bullet hits the skull with enough strength to send a piece of bone into the cranium, which can be life-threatening.

Shotgun Wounds

Shotguns fire bullets that contain a great number of small pellets. After the bullet leaves the shotgun's barrel, the pellets shoot out of the bullet and spread towards their target. This means that the further away these bullets are from the patient, the wider the affected area. A shotgun wound at contact produces a single wound on the entrance, but a spread and irregular exit wound. Close-range shotgun wounds are spread larger as the range increases. These entrance wounds can get from a central round wound with several smaller circular wounds around it to a larger number of individual holes with a defused entrance wound at the center.

Shotgun wounds are very dangerous at short range because of their great deformation capacity; however, they become less dangerous as the range increases. These, however, are much harder to treat without specialized equipment and trained personal.

Assessment and Treatment

A fast evaluation of gunshot wounds is necessary to predict the possible damage to the patient and set a treatment plan. By understanding the basic anatomy, the clinician knows which structures the bullet can harm. Also, basic understanding ballistics will tell the clinician the possible extension of the damage, as well as the chance that the bullet changed direction radically inside the patient's body. It's necessary to understand this before attempting to heal the patient's gunshot wounds.

Chapter 5

Cardiopulmonary Resuscitation

S ome patients are in more serious conditions than others. Depending on how much time it takes to treat them, how much blood they lose during the transportation, or many other different factors, a patient's breathing could stop, or worse, his breathing and his heartbeats. These patients are going through cardiopulmonary arrest, are in immediate danger, and require cardiopulmonary resuscitation as soon as possible.

Cardiopulmonary resuscitation (or CPR) is a lifesaving technique. It's used for cardiopulmonary arrest, drowning patients, even heart attacks. When the heart stops, a person can die within eight or ten minutes because of the lack of oxygenated blood to the brain. The idea is that, if the heart is unable to beat on its own, then the paramedic must help the heart pump mechanically until more advanced methods and treatments are available to the patients, or until clinical death has been declared by a professional.

Follow the DRS

There are a couple of simple steps you must take before practicing CPR on a patient. This is especially relevant for situations in which you find the patient lying on the ground, and you believe he needs CPR. You must assess the general situation, check whether the patient's conscious or not, and ask for help.

Danger

D is for danger in the DRS system. The first thing you, or any paramedic, should do as soon as you get to the scene is check whether there's any danger for you or the patient. If the traumatized patient is located near a car accident, in the middle of a road, close to a wildfire, or in any other dire circumstances, getting him out of danger goes before anything else.

Response

Assess the patient's condition by talking to him. This is an excellent moment to assess the Glasgow Coma Scale (more details in chapter seven). By measuring the Glasgow Coma Scale, you'll have a clear idea of the patient's mental condition and whether there may be a brain injury or not.

Scream for Help

Seek help from those around you and make sure that professional help is on its way. Since you're going to take charge of performing the CPR, ask someone else to call an ambulance. If the CPR isn't enough to restart the patient's heartbeats, you must do CPR until professional help arrives. You must make sure that's going to happen as soon as possible. There's a special device called an Automatic External Defibrillator (or AED). These devices deliver electric currents to patients under cardiorespiratory arrest, aiming to restore the heartbeat. They come with instructions, and they don't need any special training to use them. Larger commerce's and businesses usually have one of those available, so if there is one close to you, you should ask someone else to look for it and get it as soon as possible.

Follow the CAB

Once you've covered the DRS, it's time to start cardiopulmonary resuscitation.

Compressions

This is the first step of the CPR. The clinician kneels next to the patient and pushes down on his sternum to help his heart breathe mechanically and restore the blood flow.

- First of all, the patient must be placed over a flat surface. If the patient's lying over a bed, couch, or anything else able to bounce back during the compressions, these won't be as effective or get the necessary effect.

- Secondly, the paramedic must get on a comfortable kneeling position next to the patient. If he's right-handed, he should kneel to the patient's right side and stay as close as possible. If he's left-handed, he must kneel to the patient's left side. In any case, the clinician must get as close to the patient's chest and head as possible.

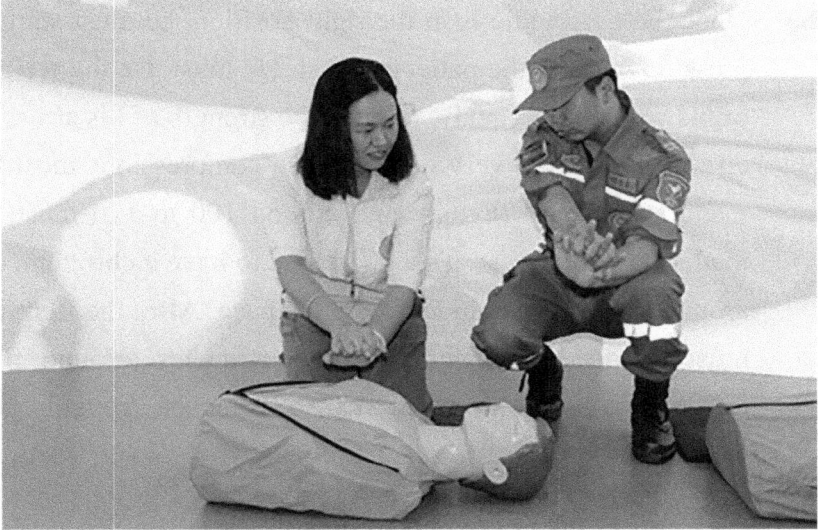

- Next, the clinician must place the heel of one of his hands over the patient's sternum at about the height of his nipples. The other hand must be placed over the first one, and then the clinician has to lean forward over the patient until his shoulders are aligned with his hands.

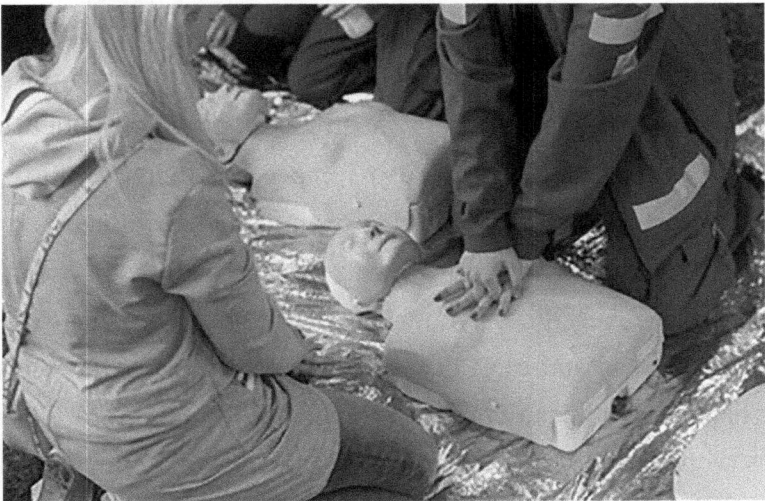

- Once the paramedic is in the right position, he must start to press down over the patient's chest. He must use the weight of his whole upper body, not just the strength of his arms, or else he'll get tired very quickly. The compressions must be made at a steady rhythm, and around 100 to 120 must be made each minute, so it's a good idea to have a chronometer around to help the clinician keep the pace. Also, the sternum must be pressed down at least two inches (around five centimeters), but no more than 2.4 inches (roughly six centimeters).

- Count until you have made thirty compressions and move forward with the next step. The American Heart Association recommends keeping with the chest compressions if you're not trained in CPR. So it's highly advisable to practice the next steps thoroughly to make sure you're doing them correctly.

Airway

The compressions are intended to replace the natural heartbeats, but that's not the only problem. If the heart has stopped, the patient's not breathing either, so we must also replace the lungs to allow the patient to survive. But first, the airways must be positioned in a way that favors breathing and airflow; this is done with the head-tilt and chin-lift maneuver. First, you have to place your hand over the patient's forehead and carefully push it back; then, you'll place your other hand under the patient's chin and gently lift it forward. The idea is to straighten the pharynx, larynx, and trachea to facilitate airflow;

however, this must be done carefully because you don't want to move a traumatized patient's neck too much, in case there's an injury to the cervical vertebrae.

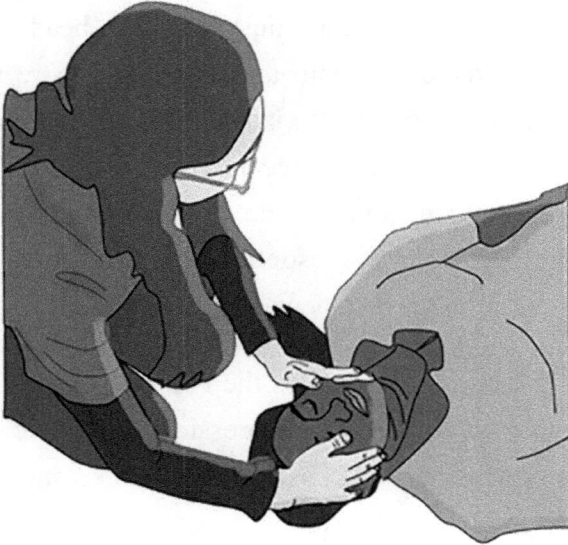

Breathing

Once the airways are opened, the patient's ready to receive mouth-to-mouth or mouth-to-nose breathing. Mouth-to-mouth is the preferred method, but if the patient's mouth is injured or unable to open, the clinician has to use mouth-to-nose.

- The clinician must close the patient's nostrils by squeezing his nose with his fingers before providing the rescue breath. Then, he must take air in and cover the patient's mouth with his own, making a seal.

- The clinician lets the air go into the patient's mouth for the duration of one second, that's the first rescue breath. He checks to see if the patient's chest rises. If it rises, that means the air is going into his lungs; however, if the patient's chest doesn't rise, the clinician must apply the head-tilt and chin-lift maneuver once again and do it one more time. If the abdomen is the one rising instead of the chest, then the air's probably running down the pharynx, esophagus, and then stomach. This means that the clinician is blowing too hard. Blowing air into the esophagus can provoke a stomach perforation, which is a dangerous complication of the CPR.

- Once the clinician provides the two rescue breaths, he must go back to the chest compressions. A cycle of CPR is composed of thirty chest compressions and two rescue breaths.

- If an automatic external defibrillator is ever available, all the clinician must do is follow the device's instructions. The AED will provide one shock; then, the clinician must restore CPR for two more minutes until the AED provides a second shock. If the instructions aren't clear, any 911 operator will be able to provide real-time instructions through the phone until the professional paramedics arrive or the patient is transported to a health facility. The main function of the AED is to restore the heart's electrical activity to normal, especially fibrillations. These are a particular kind of tachyarrhythmia so fast that it doesn't allow the heart to beat. They also provide an EKG reading with an automatic diagnosis; this way, the clinician is capable of knowing what's going on with the heart's electrical activity, and whether there's an arrhythmia or a lack of electrical stimuli (asystole), without the knowledge of how to read an EKG.

- If an AED is not available, the clinician must keep with the CPR cycle until there's professional help ready to take over the patient's treatment, or the patient starts breathing again.

The Value of Teamwork

If you're the only one available around a person in need of CPR, there's no way around it. However, the chances are that there'll be at least someone else around, and this can make things much easier. Besides asking someone else to take care of everything else while you're stuck with the CPR cycles, you can also ask for help with the CPR itself. If there's another person trained with CPR, the best way to work together is by having one of you do the compressions, and the other one does the breathing. Whoever is doing the compressions can also do the head-tilt and chin-lift maneuver, and keep the head in that position, so the other one has an easier job. Both of you can also switch positions if the one doing the compressions gets tired.

Breathing CPR

If the patient's heart is beating, but he's still not breathing, the patient won't need the compressions, but he'll still need help breathing to sustain his life. The clinician must open the airways using the head-tilt and chin-lift maneuver, and then he'll follow the steps to give the patient mouth-to-mouth or mouth-to-nose breathing. The clinician must give one rescue breath every five or six seconds to keep the patient alive until he starts breathing again, or there's more help coming..

Gunshot Injured Patients

There are many other things we must do with patients who've suffered a gunshot wound. Bleeding must be stopped, injuries, and conditions must be assessed, and the patient must be kept alive by any means available until transport is available to an adequate health facility. If you're treating a patient with a gunshot wound and he goes into cardiorespiratory arrest, restoring the patient's heartbeat must be prioritized over everything else. This doesn't mean that you should stop the compression that you're using to stop the bleeding. In these cases, you should use the help of anyone else available to maintain the pressure over the gunshot wound while you perform CPR. However, if you're on your own, cardiopulmonary resuscitation is more important to save the patient's life, and it must be practiced by all means.

The technique of cardiopulmonary resuscitation will be useful to you in other situations. Once you understand how to do this, your help's not limited to gunshot patients, but drowned patients and those who're suffering from heart attacks. Follow the steps, practice them at home, and you'll know how to save a life or at least sustain it until there's more specialized treatment on the way.

Note: If you're in a life-threatening or emergency medical situation, seek medical assistance immediately.

Chapter 6

Bandages and Transportation

M ost deaths due to gunshot wounds are because of massive bleeding. The following cause is a tension pneumothorax caused by penetrating wounds to the chest. Learning about bandages and how to use them correctly is the only way to treat these conditions in an emergency scenario. Also, before any patient is ready to be transported to a health center, he must be immobilized. Professional paramedics will take care of this once they arrive at the scene. However, if you're the one who has to transport the patient, then you must learn about immobilizations.

Types of Bandages by Material

The first step to learn how to use a bandage is to know what the different bandages are good for.

Gauze Bandages

These are the most common kind of bandages, and they're also the most used ones. They're made of a woven fabric, and they're sterilized and packaged to be used later. These are the bandages that we use to put pressure on the bleeding wounds. They're also used to clean wounds and to disinfect the skin before and after applying injections. They're clean, easy to handle, and they have a high capacity to absorb fluids.

Compression Bandages

These are the bandages used to apply pressure, immobilize the patient, improve circulation, and make improvised tourniquets. They're stronger than gauzes, but they don't have the same capacity to absorb fluids, so they're not fit to absorb the bleeding. However, they have many other uses. If you don't have a specialized bandage for immobilizations at hand, these are the bandages you should use to prepare a patient for transportation.

Triangular Bandages

These are specialized bandages used for immobilizations in the arms, forearms, and shoulders. They're strong bandages shaped like a right-angled triangle; the tip of this angle is called the apex of the bandage. Their shape and resistance make them comfortable for a splint, as well as other uses.

Tube Bandages

As the name implies, these are elastic bandages shaped like a tube. They're fabricated like this so we can squeeze them around limbs, even fingers; this way, we can hold objects towards a patient's extremities for stability, such as splints. They make the process of immobilization much easier.

Specialized Bandages

In the treatment and management of gunshot wounds, there are two types of bandages that deserve a special mention. These are chest seals and combat gauzes. Combat gauzes work like normal gauzes, with the difference that they're covered with chemical agents that improve clot-formation and help to stop the bleeding. Chest seals are also similar to gauzes in the way that they're used directly over the wound, but they're harder and more resistant. Chest seals are more solid because they're used to cover penetrating wounds to the chest, avoiding air to enter the pleural cavity. One of the borders of a chest seal is usually a flutter valve to allow the air to come out.

Application of Bandages

Once you've learned about the types of bandages and what they're used for, it's important to understand how to use them.

Wound Pressure

This is the first step to stop the bleeding. The clinician uses gauze bandages to put pressure over the bleeding wound. The pressure must be strong enough to stop the bleeding, so it's advised to use the palms of the hands instead of the fingertips to press the gauze towards the bleeding. Small wounds with mild bleeding might only need wound pressure, but larger wounds will need other measures depending on their location.

Wound Packing

This is a technique used to stop large bleeding wounds. The clinician fills the wound with gauze bandages and covers them to make a seal.

This improves clot-formation, stopping the bleeding at once. This is exactly where clinicians with a basic knowledge of anatomy get their knowledge to practice. By studying the type of bleeding and the location of the wound, they have an idea of the ruptured blood vessel and the direction at which they should point the gauze bandages. Arterial bleeding wounds need the gauzes to be pointed in a proximal direction since that's where the blood of the arteries comes from. By contrast, a venous bleeding wound needs gauzes to be pointed in the opposite direction since that's where the blood of the vein comes from. Also, knowledge of the type of bullet, firearm, and distance from the shot will tell the clinician the expected damage around the wound, as well as the direction he should cover with the gauze bandages if he finds an exit wound. The location of the large blood vessels that could have been damaged by the bullet tells the clinician where to point the gauze bandages.

The first gauzes are going to get completely soaked with blood. This is normal, and it's what we're looking for. You can't take these gauzes out of the wound, or else the process of clot-formation will be stopped, and the bleeding will start again. All you need to do is attach a gauze bandage directly to the wounded vessel. After the first gauzes have been placed, the rest of the wound must be packed and covered with them. Once that's done, the clinician must apply pressure for at least three minutes. The packing of the wound is finished by attaching the bandages towards the wound with a compression bandage. Sometimes you can place a splint with the compression bandage to avoid the packing to be undone during the transport of the patient.

Tourniquets

Tourniquets are strong bandages designed to be tied around a limb and to stop blood flow towards it completely. Since they're very constricting and don't allow blood to reach the limb, they're the *last resource in the treatment of an uncontrollable bleeding wound.* Whenever wound pressure and wound packing are enough to stop the bleeding, do NOT use a tourniquet.

Blood deprivation can be lethal to tissues, and if a tissue spends too much time without receiving blood, necrosis can overcome. Besides this, tourniquets are only fit to be applied at limbs. You can't stop bleeding from the neck or torso with a tourniquet.

The location of the tourniquet is also extremely important. Tourniquets must be placed at least two inches above the wound. In order to stop the bleeding, we need to cut the blood flow of the artery. This is also true for venous bleeding because veins usually run deeper than arteries, so it's very difficult to stop venous bleeding with a tourniquet. Also, tourniquets shouldn't be placed over joints. If the bleeding is right below the elbow or the wrist, the tourniquet has to be above those joints and never directly over it.

There are many different commercial tourniquets, and you should have at least one of them available in your first aid kit. These work better and are highly advisable for any emergencies. Some tourniquets have inflation pumps, just like the sphygmomanometer, and use them to stop the bleeding. Other tourniquets are just a belt with a strap to minimize the required force to squeeze them around the limbs. However, if you don't have a commercial tourniquet at hand, you'll have to use an improvised tourniquet. Compression bandages, cloth, belts, even towels can be used as a tourniquet if that's what you have available at the moment. Place the cloth material around the limb, tie it with a simple square knot (the first one you use on your shoelaces before you finish it) and squeeze it hard. If you're not strong enough to stop the bleeding, or if you can't tie the tourniquet in a way that it stops relying on your strength to remain in its place, you can use a stick to help you with the tourniquet. These sticks can be made of wood, metal tubes, even plastic tubes if that's what you have at hand. The only requirement is that they're resistant and have the right size. Once you find a stick, you must place it over the square knot of the tourniquet and tie a second knot around it. Then you must start spinning the stick in a clockwise direction to squeeze the tourniquet harder around the limb.

It's important to point out that tourniquets are extremely painful and uncomfortable. If applied correctly, a conscious patient could even beg for its removal. However, this is exactly the way a tourniquet should be applied; it doesn't work unless it stops the bleeding correctly. Tourniquets are temporary solutions because if they're left for too long over the limb, they'll harm the tissue below it. However, if everything else fails, it's better to lose a leg than to lose a life.

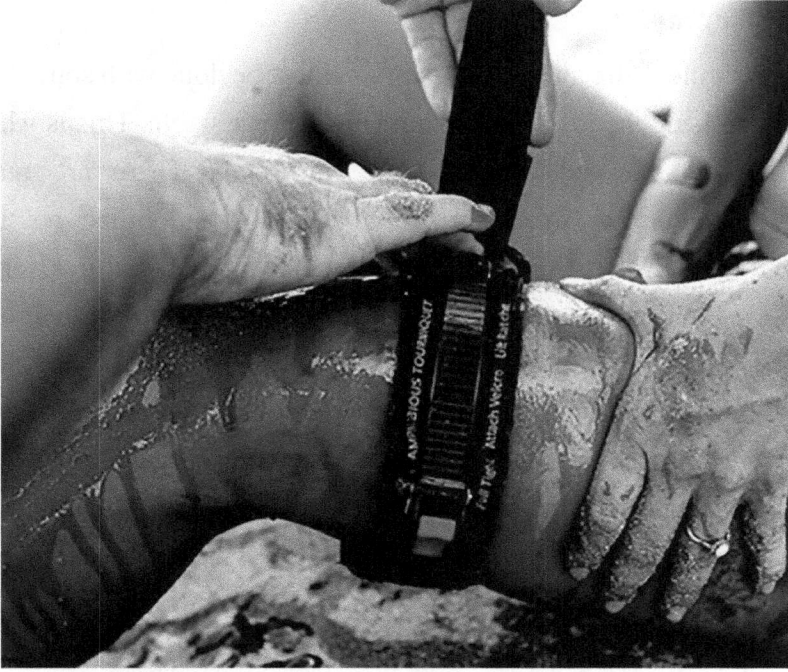

Rules for Immobilizations

When we suspect a fracture, we can't allow the patient to be transported without proper immobilization, or else there's a high risk that the fracture will get worse. The involved bones could grow further from each other, making it more difficult to treat and recover the fracture, and the bone fragments can damage the surrounding tissue. Also, any traumatized patient who may have received a blow to the head or the neck should have his neck immobilized. The cervical vertebrae are very weak, and injuries to the spinal cord are very dangerous, especially in that area (more details in chapter two). So applying a neck immobilization is standard for traumatized patients. There are three main rules to apply any immobilization technique correctly.

Look for Stability

The first rule is that the immobilization must be done with something strong to keep the affected anatomical segment stable. This is where splints and cervical collars come into play. There are many commercial splints intended to be used to immobilize possible fractures, such as radius and ulna fractures, humerus fractures, femur fractures, and else. Some of these commercial splints have their own belts and straps to be held against the fractured bone. Other splints need the help of another kind of support, such as a compression bandage or a tube bandage, to be tied around the affected limb. If you don't have a commercial splint, you may use anything suitable as an improvised splint that you have at hand. You can use sticks, planks, shoes, even cardboard if it's resistant enough, and you find a large amount of it. Improvised splints must be adapted to the anatomical shape of the affected body's segment as tightly as possible and held with a compression bandage (or anything else available) in order to work.

If you don't have anything else at hand to be used as a splint, you can use the body of the patient. You must attach two adjacent body segments, such as legs, so you make the immobilization by attaching the fractured leg to the healthy leg with a compression bandage. You can also use the patient's torso to immobilize his arms, using a triangular bandage in these cases. There are no anatomical structures adjacent to the neck, so the patient will always need any sort of object as a splint. Finding a splint to immobilize the neck is, however, simple enough. If you don't have a neck collar available, a pair of hats around the neck and a compression bandage is good enough. If there are no hats available either, a pair of shoes tied around the neck is also a good fit for those immobilizations.

Secure the Joints

The second rule for immobilization applies to limb fractures, and it's to immobilize the proximal and the distal joint to the fracture. If you want to avoid the movements in the arm, for example, you must immobilize the shoulder and the elbow. In order to immobilize the forearm, if you suspect a fractured radius or ulna, you must immobilize the elbow and the wrist. Some commercial splints are capable of adapting to the shape of the wrist, while others demand more materials to be used in order to immobilize these joints correctly. Keep in mind that all you need to do is get the limb stable enough for transportation; definitive treatment will be provided at the health center.

Not too Tight

Immobilizations must be tight enough to avoid any movements, but they can't be so tight that they change the direction of the bones, or worse, compromise circulation or airflow. The clinician must be sure that the immobilized limb isn't turning pale or blue; this would mean that circulation is compromised. For cervical spine immobilizations, squeezing too tight will also affect the neck's direction, and if the patient's having trouble breathing, or if you see that his face is turning pale or blue, that probably means you're either compromising airflow or circulation to the head.

Immobilizations According to the Segment of the Body

The body has different shapes and resting positions, and the immobilizations must adapt to these circumstances. Immobilizing an arm and a leg is not the same, so the techniques to apply these immobilizations must be studied separately.

Cervical Spine Immobilization

The most important immobilization is the cervical spine immobilization. Almost any patient will have a neck immobilization before he's transported to a health center. Placing a cervical collar is the best way to make sure the patient's cervical spine is safe. They're reliable and easy to use, so it's highly suggested to have one in the first aid kit. If you don't have a cervical collar or any other commercial neck immobilizers, cardboard, pillows, or anything else that may adjust to the shape of the neck without forcing it to tilt forward or rotate to either side.

The process of placing a cervical spine immobilization is very delicate, and it requires more than one pair of hands. One of the paramedics must lift the head and shoulders of the patient at the same time. He must lift them slowly, making sure to keep the neck in its current position. The other paramedic must place any needed immobilizer around the neck while it's lifted from the ground. Once this is in place, the patient can be put down on the ground. Then the immobilizer should be secured with straps (if it's a commercial immobilizer) or by making a knot with the previously placed compression bandage (if it's an improvised immobilizer).

Arm Immobilizers

Arm fractures are extremely common, especially radius and ulna fractures. There's no easy way to tell whether a bone is fractured or not unless you have specialized training. In the case of a gunshot wound patient, wounds in the arms could fracture bones, and they should always be treated as fractures until proven otherwise. There are two main resources used on the immobilization of an arm; these are splints and slings.

Splints are attached to the injured segment of the arm to prevent it from moving. They should also try to immobilize the proximal and distal joints of the affected segment as well as possible. Commercial splints are great for support, but any other hard materials can be used if there are no commercial splints available. The arm should always be immobilized with the elbow bent in a ninety degrees angle (for upper arm injuries) or tighter angle (for lower arm injuries), so the splint must be adapted to meet the bent arm. Hard and malleable materials such as cardboard are ideal because they can be bent easily.

Once the splint is placed, the next step is to use a sling. Slings are useful for any possible fractures in the arm, no matter the location. They immobilize the arms, bring stability, and even help with the bleeding depending on the location. There are three types of slings you should learn and understand in order to treat gunshot wound patients; the two first ones need a triangular bandage or a triangular or rectangular sheet of clothing that could be adapted as one, the third one's meant to be used if there's no triangular bandage available.

Arm slings are the most common. Their main focus is to immobilize the upper arm, so they're great for shoulder, humerus, clavicle, and even rib immobilization if there's a suspected fracture in the thoracic cage. The process of placing an arm sling begins by placing the triangular bandage under the arm with the apex of the bandage pointing at the elbow, the shorter side pointing at the healthy shoulder, and the longer side facing towards the feet. Once the bandage is in the right position, the top side is taken behind the neck and towards the damaged shoulder. Then the longer side is taken up, over the patient's forearm, and to the damaged shoulder where it meets the tip of the shorter side of the bandage. Both tips are tied together, and the corners of the knot are tucked down below the bandage. By this point, the arm and forearm should be already in the right position, with the forearm placed horizontally with a slight elevation towards the hand. The sling is finished by extending the bandage towards the little finger, providing support to the arm all the way to the fingertips. Then the apex of the bandage is tied behind the elbow to improve stability.

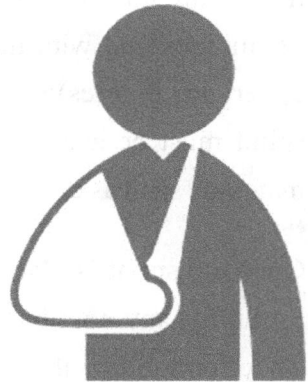

The second kind of sling is the elevated arm sling. These slings are best for the lower arm, so they're used in forearm, wrist, and hand injuries. Since they elevate the forearm towards the healthy shoulder, they're great at reducing forearm and hand bleeding. The process of applying an elevated hand sling begins by placing the injured forearm diagonally over the chest, with the fingertips over the healthy shoulder. Then the triangular bandage is placed over the arm with one end over the healthy shoulder and the apex over the elbow. The lower edge of the bandage is then tucked under the forearm and the elbow. The free end of the bandage is taken behind the patient's back and directed diagonally towards the healthy elbow to meet the other end (remember to be careful with the immobilization of the cervical and thoracic spine). Both ends of the bandage are tied together, and the corners of the knot are tucked under the bandage. Then the apex of the bandage is tied shut to improve the stability behind the elbow.

The last type of sling is the collar-and-cuff sling. It doesn't provide as much stability and comfort as the other ones, but it's the only resource available if there are no triangular bandages. It uses a compression bandage or any sort of cloth that can be folded until it resembles a compression bandage. The center of the compression bandage is placed behind the patient's neck and healthy shoulder, with both ends of the bandage pointing down towards the arm. Depending on whether you want to prioritize the upper arm and elbow (arm sling), or the lower arm (elevated arm sling), place the arm in the desired position. Once the arm is in place, the sling is finished by tying a knot above the wrist, taking both tips around the wrist, and tying a knot below it.

After finishing the immobilization of the arm, it's important to assess the circulation in order to make sure the sling or the splint does not compromise it. The way to assess circulation is by squeezing one of the fingertips of the affected arm. The fingertip should turn pale under the pressure because it's no longer receiving blood. If the fingertip recovers its color in under three seconds after the pressure's released, then there's no compromise in the circulation of the arm; if it doesn't, then immobilization should be assessed and done again. Of course, if there's massive blood loss or a tourniquet placed on the arm, circulation assessment is impossible.

Leg Immobilization

In an emergency, immobilizing a leg is less complicated than immobilizing an arm. Also, since the bones in the leg are stronger, it's less likely that they'll get fractured by a bullet. Most leg splints are used to relieve strains. However, it's still valuable to learn how to immobilize a leg correctly.

The knee joint should be slightly flexed. The patient's leg can't be completely straight during immobilization, but it can't be too flexed either. Sometimes it helps to place a small roll of bandage under the knee to allow this slight flexion to take place. When it comes to the ankle, the angle between the leg and the foot should be of ninety degrees. Most commercial leg splints already come prepared to keep the foot in the right position, but if the paramedic doesn't have one available, adapting a splint to the back of the leg should be enough to get the desired effect. These immobilizations also use compression bandages to keep the splint attached to the leg. Remember that you can use the healthy as a splint for the injured leg. The paramedic should also check the circulation of the leg to be sure it's not compromised by squeezing it gently.

Thoracic and Lumbar Spine Immobilization

The neck can be immobilized with a splint, but there's no splint big enough to immobilize the thoracic or lumbar spines. Both of these anatomical structures also protect a segment of the spinal cord, so whenever we suspect damage to these structures, they must be treated carefully. They may not be as fragile as the cervical spine, but they're still vulnerable to trauma, and injuries to the spinal cord are unable to heal and recover.

Professional paramedics will carry around a stretcher and apply the correct transport techniques to immobilize the whole spine. The stretcher will be lowered until it's right next to the patient's body to avoid injuries when the patient is located over it. Then they work in groups to lift the patient and place him over the stretcher, making sure to avoid any flexions and rotations of the spine. Once the patient is in the stretcher, he's secured with straps to keep his torso from rotating, flexing and extending. That's the last step of the immobilization before getting the patient into the ambulance and transporting him to a health center.

If you're on your own, you probably won't have a stretcher at hand. You should wait for professional paramedics to take over the immobilization and transportation of the patient. However, if you know they're not coming, and you must take charge of the transportation yourself, you should make your best effort to avoid thoracic and lumbar spine movements. When you get ready to lift the patient to the vehicle you'll use for transportation, ask for help. If you have one person lifting the head and shoulders, one or two more helpers lifting the torso, and one last helper lifting the legs by the ankles, you should be able to move the patient while keeping spine movements to a minimum. If there's nobody else to give you a hand, you must make do with what you have. Carrying the patient over your back or dragging him by the legs is a valid alternative if there's no other way to get the patient to a specialized health center. Remember that this is the last step of the process of immobilization. Cervical spine immobilization is *prior* to thoracic and lumbar spine immobilization, and other required limb immobilizations and splints should be in place before lifting the patient.

Note: If you're in a life-threatening or emergency medical situation, seek medical assistance immediately.

Chapter 7

Vital Signs and Other Measurements

Initial Assessment

The first thing every clinician must do to treat an injured patient is to run a complete assessment. This assessment must be done as quickly as possible; it has a predesigned order to follow that's been proven to improve the patient's possibilities for recovery, and it must be done correctly. Paramedics do three main things whenever they deal with a patient in a prehospital setting. They run the assessment, they stabilize the patient, and they notify the health center to coordinate the hospital treatment. This communication is absolutely vital because it allows the health center to mobilize the personnel and get ready to receive the patient. Also, time in the scene before transporting the patient to a hospital must be as short as possible, especially for critical patients.

The first step of the initial assessment is to take vital signs. Vital signs are indicators that show us the most basic body functions; this the fastest way to assess the condition of a traumatized patient. In the ATLS system, prehospital staff should focus first on the respiratory rate, systolic blood pressure, and the Glasgow Coma Scale. After these are measured, the clinician can focus on the pulse rate and other vital information that will be valuable for the hospital staff. Taking these measurements shouldn't take more than ninety seconds, even sixty seconds for trained professionals. Fast measurements save lives, and the health professionals know that. If you want to help someone and make sure you save a life, you must practice taking these signs at home until you're proficient enough with them.

Respiratory Rate

This is the measure of the breaths per minute. Patients under physical or mental stress can show an increase in the respiratory rate. This is an autonomic response of the nervous system intended to secure the oxygen supply to the body, especially to the brain. When the nervous system, as well as the rest of the systems, are shutting down, the respiratory rate can go the other way and will be under normal rates. This happens when the patient reaches a critical condition, and it's a sign of alarm. The normal respiratory rate should be between 12 and 20 breaths per minute. Higher than that is called tachypnea, and lower than that is considered bradypnea. For the ATLS, patients with tachypnea higher than 29 breaths per minute, as well as patients with bradypnea lower than ten breaths per minute, should be taken immediately to an advanced trauma facility.

Measuring the Respiratory Rate

In order to measure the respiratory rate, the patient must be unaware of what's going on. A conscious patient can't be aware of this measure, or else he may distort the reading by accelerating or decelerating his breathing. So you have to make sure the patient doesn't realize what you're doing. Breathing is observed through the movements of the thorax and abdomen, particularly the expansion of the chest, abdomen, and movement of the shoulders. If a patient's breathing is too shallow to perceive, you can aid yourself by placing your hand over the abdomen to feel its ascension. You can do this while also placing your head on the patient's chest to listen to the breathing and heartbeats. This last maneuver will allow you to measure the heart rate, which is another vital sign that's invaluable for the medical team waiting at the hospital.

Regarding the part of counting breaths, this must be done using a chronometer. You could count the number of breaths for one minute. This is the most reliable way to assess the respiratory rate, but during an emergency, spending a whole minute with the respiratory-rate measurement is a waste of time. As long as the breathing is steady and regular, you can count the number of breaths for thirty seconds and multiply that by two to get the respiratory rate. You could even count them for twenty seconds and multiply that by three. The only valid reason to waste sixty seconds measuring the respiratory rate is if this is irregular. If you realize that the patient's breathing accelerates and decelerates constantly, you can't predict the respiratory rate with a twenty or thirty seconds measure.

Systolic Blood Pressure

The systolic blood pressure is the force produced by the impact of the blood when it's running through your arteries. It's the force of the blood when it's running through our arteries. Blood pressure isn't a vital sign; however, it's always measured on critical patients. On a physiological and physical level, it's the resistance of the arteries against the upcoming blood flow. It's a measure of the strength of the heart, as well as the resistance of your arteries. Measuring blood pressure needs specialized equipment. If you wish to be able to help someone who received a gunshot wound, you must always have a blood pressure monitor around you in case you ever need it.

Blood pressure is divided into two measures. There's the systolic blood pressure, which we've already explained, and the diastolic blood pressure, which is the force produced by the blood flowing back to the heart. When we speak about the diastolic blood pressure from a physiological and physical perspective, it's the resistance of the heart against the blood flowing back to it. As much as this is relevant for the general health of a patient, it's not so vital for emergencies. In the initial assessment of an injured patient, the systolic blood pressure will tell us what we need to know about his condition.

The Measurement Procedure

Measuring the systolic blood pressure is a lot easier and faster when you use an automatic blood pressure monitor. There are small devices that you can strap to the arm or wrist of the patient, and they'll give you the measurements you're looking for.

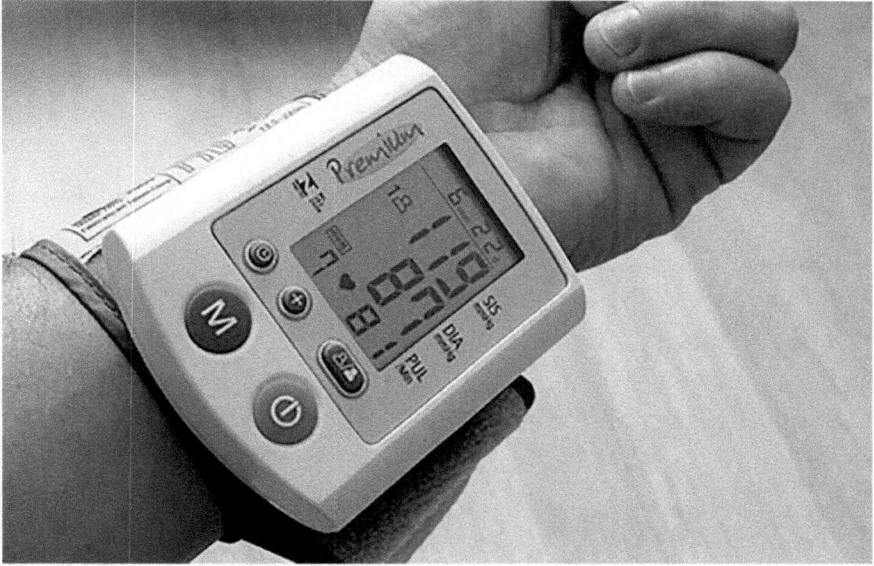

Blood pressure is recorded as "mmHg" (millimeters of mercury). The higher value will be the systolic blood pressure; this is considered normal between 90 mmHg and 120 mmHg. A value higher than that tells us of systolic hypertension, which is a very serious medical condition, but it's not what we're concerned about when we face a traumatized patient. Systolic hypotension, a value below 90 mmHg of systolic blood pressure, is the real reason to worry about a gunshot wounded patient. This happens when there's significant blood loss or an injury to the heart. Systolic hypotension is a reason to transfer the patient immediately to a trauma center.

The blood pressure monitor will also give you the diastolic blood pressure. This value should be between 60 mmHg and 90 mmHg. In a traumatized patient, the diastolic blood pressure will be the last one to be affected by the blood loss, so it's not used as an immediate reference to assess the patient's status. Most automatic blood pressure monitors will also give you the pulse rate of the patient, which is the lower number that you see in the picture. This is relevant, and we will cover this later in the book.

When you start getting items for your first aid kit, you should always get an automatic blood pressure monitor. However, if all you have available is a manual sphygmomanometer, you should also know how to use this in order to get the measurement you need.

First of all, a manual sphygmomanometer looks like this:

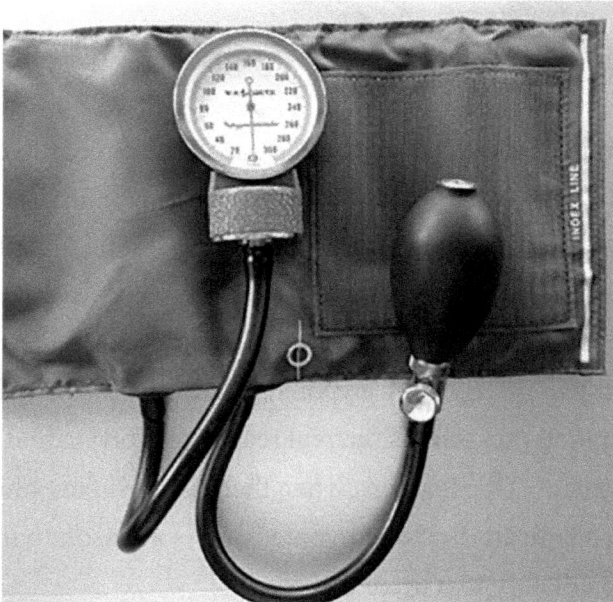

The larger part of the sphygmomanometer is the cuff; it's the part that is wrapped around the arm of the patient. The round and black part is the inflation bulb; you must squeeze it to fill the cuff with air and press the arm's arteries. The small round silver valve right next to the inflation bulb is the air releasing valve; this controls the air output of the cuff. When it's closed, it doesn't allow air to leave the cuff, and when it's slightly opened, it allows the air to leave gradually. The round piece with a gauge is the aneroid manometer gauge. It has a needle that points at the current pressure in the cuff, measured in mmHg. Unless you're extremely proficient at taking the pulse with your fingers, you'll need to use a stethoscope with the sphygmomanometer to measure blood pressure.

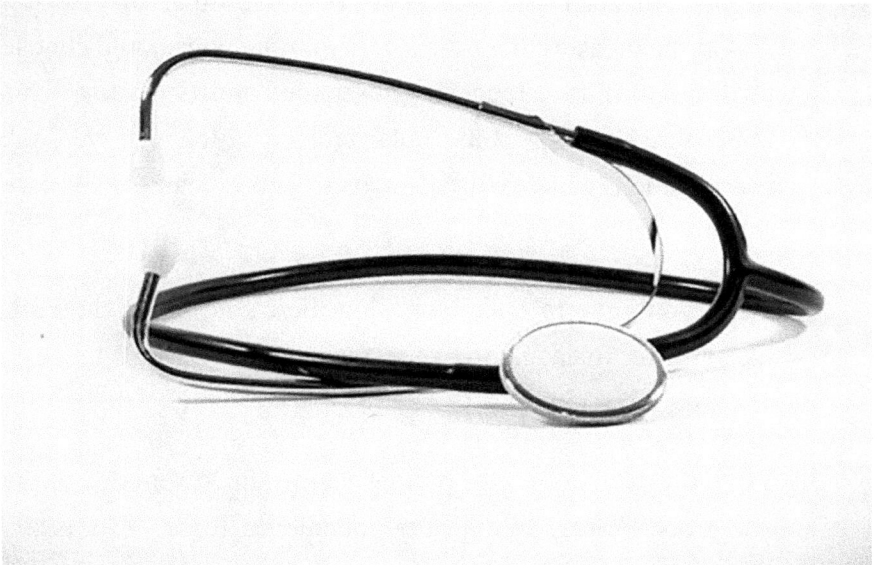

You've probably seen health professionals using them many times. The round piece is called a diaphragm, and it goes over the body surface you wish to hear. The two white pieces located at the other end are the earpieces. They go inside your ears to allow you to listen, in this case, to the sounds of the blood flowing.

Some sphygmomanometers have an integrated stethoscope. Those sphygmomanometers have the diaphragm integrated into the cuff, and the earpieces are free at the other end so you can plug them into your ears and measure blood pressure comfortably.

The procedure to measure blood pressure isn't hard at all. It may take a little practice at first, but once you dominate it, it'll come as easy as riding a bicycle.

1. First, you must uncover the arm you wish to take the measure from. You can't place the cuff over clothing, or else it'll distort the measurement. As a general rule, you should choose the left arm if the patient is right-handed and vice-versa. This is because there's less muscular tension in the arm we don't use as much, which will allow us to get a cleaner and more reliable reading.

2. Next, you have to make sure that there's no air in the cuff. Open the air releasing the valve and squeeze the cuff to let go of all the air remaining.

3. Wrap the cuff around the patient's arm. The lower edge of the cuff must be higher than the antecubital fossa. This is the opposite face of the elbow; the division between the biceps and the forearm.

4. Place the stethoscope's diaphragm over the antecubital fossa, slightly over the cuff's lower edge. The brachial artery runs under the antecubital fossa, which is the reason why we measure blood pressure there.

5. Close the air releasing valve, put on the earpieces, stare directly at the manometer, and inflate the cuff until the

manometer's needle reaches 180 mmHg. This is done by repeatedly squeezing the sphygmomanometer's inflation bulb.

6. The number marked me the manometer corresponds with the pressure we've placed over the patient's arm. Once the needle reaches 180 mmHg, slightly open the air releasing valve so that the pressure starts to drop slowly. It should drop down at a rate of around three mmHg per second to make sure that you take the right measurement. By using the stethoscope, you shall hear a knocking sound once the pressure goes under the patient's systolic blood pressure. This first knocking sound is called the "korotkoff" sound. With that sound, you'll start to hear the blood flowing in rhythmical knocking sounds. When you stop hearing the knocking sounds, that means you've reached the patient's diastolic blood pressure, so pay attention to the manometer's lowering needle.

7. Take note of the mmHg value in which you heard the korotkoff sound, that's the value of the systolic blood pressure. Take also note of the diastolic blood pressure, which corresponds to the mmHg value when you stopped listening to the rhythmical knocking sounds.

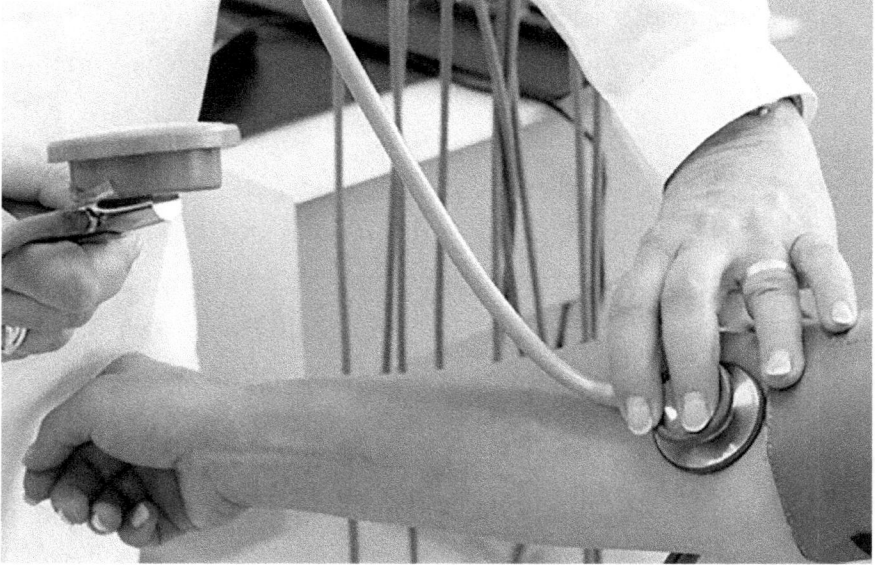

You've probably seen health professionals using them many times. The round piece is called a diaphragm, and it goes over the body surface you wish to hear. The two white pieces located at the other end are the earpieces. They go inside your ears to allow you to listen, in this case, to the sounds of the blood flowing.

Some sphygmomanometers have an integrated stethoscope. Those sphygmomanometers have the diaphragm integrated into the cuff, and the earpieces are free at the other end so you can plug them into your ears and measure blood pressure comfortably.

The procedure to measure blood pressure isn't hard at all. It may take a little practice at first, but once you dominate it, it'll come as easy as riding a bicycle.

1. First of all, you must uncover the arm you wish to take the measure from. You can't place the cuff over clothing, or else it'll distort the measurement. As a general rule, you should choose the left arm if the patient is right-handed and vice-versa. This is because there's less muscular tension in the arm we don't use as much, which will allow us to get a cleaner and more reliable reading.

2. Next, you have to make sure that there's no air in the cuff. Open the air releasing the valve and squeeze the cuff to let go of all the air remaining.

3. Wrap the cuff around the patient's arm. The lower edge of the cuff must be higher than the antecubital fossa. This is the opposite face of the elbow; the division between the biceps and the forearm.

4. Place the stethoscope's diaphragm over the antecubital fossa, slightly over the cuff's lower edge. The brachial artery runs under the antecubital fossa, which is the reason why we measure blood pressure there.

5. Close the air releasing valve, put on the earpieces, stare directly at the manometer, and inflate the cuff until the manometer's needle reaches 180 mmHg. This is done by repeatedly squeezing the sphygmomanometer's inflation bulb.

6. The number marked by the manometer corresponds with the pressure we've placed over the patient's arm. Once the needle reaches 180 mmHg, slightly open the air releasing valve so

that the pressure starts to drop slowly. It should drop down at a rate of around three mmHg per second to make sure that you take the right measurement. By using the stethoscope, you shall hear a knocking sound once the pressure goes under the patient's systolic blood pressure. This first knocking sound is called the "korotkoff" sound. With that sound, you'll start to hear the blood flowing in rhythmical knocking sounds. When you stop hearing the knocking sounds, that means you've reached the patient's diastolic blood pressure, so pay attention to the manometer's lowering needle.

7. Take note of the mmHg value in which you heard the korotkoff sound, that's the value of the systolic blood pressure. Take also note of the diastolic blood pressure, which corresponds to the mmHg value when you stopped listening to the rhythmical knocking sounds.

Glasgow	Coma	Scale
Eyes	Open spontaneously	+4
	Open to sound	+3
	Open to pressure	+2
	Don't open	+1
Verbal	Oriented	+5

	Confused	+4
	Inappropriate words	+3
	Incomprehensible sounds	+2
	No verbal response	+1
Motor	Obey commands	+6
	Localize pain	+5
	Normal flexion	+4
	Abnormal flexion	+3
	Extension to pain	+2
	No motor response	+1

The Glasgow Coma Scale, as mentioned earlier, derives from the observation of the patient's response to external stimuli. It's fairly simple and easy to apply, and its value to predict a patient's current state and the possible outcome makes it a vital tool. However, it may seem confusing at first sight, especially for a beginner. We're going to explain it thoroughly to leave no room for doubts.

Eyes

The eyes are expected to open spontaneously because an active mind is always aware of its surroundings. If the patient opens his eyes on his own, without needing a particular stimulus, he gets a score of +4.

If the patient has his eyes closed, and he only opens them if someone tries to speak with him, or if he is clearly listening, he gets a score of +3. The first approach to a patient usually involves speaking to him.

If the patient doesn't open his eyes when spoken to, but he answers to pain or pressure, then he gets a score of +2. This is a patient you try to speak with, he doesn't answer, and you have to squeeze one of his thumbs or press over his sternum to get him to open his eyes.

If the patient never opens his eyes, no matter what you do to him, he gets +1 on this score. This is a patient that never reacts, even to pain or pressure.

Verbal

This factor gauges the verbal response of the patient. It's also measured by speaking with the patient, so it's easy to assess. It's just a matter of learning the values of the different responses in the scale and how they present themselves.

A patient that speaks normally gets a value of +5. This is a patient that speaks in complete sentences if asked to and is not confused at all. This means that the patient understands where, when, and who he is.

A patient that shows signs of confusion, however, gets a +4 in the scale. This is a patient able to speak in complete sentences but isn't sure about where or when he is. He may be wrong about the exact date, or the place he's currently in. Sometimes these patients may even be confused about who they are. There are psychiatric illnesses able to provoke these situations, such as dementia, Alzheimer's Disease, or schizophrenia. However, when you deal with a traumatized patient, this isn't the first diagnosis you should think about, especially if there are no reasons to believe it or personal history to back that diagnosis. An injured patient that's confused is most likely taking an injure to the central nervous system.

If a patient is unable to speak in complete sentences, but he's capable of vocalizing words, he is given a +3. These words are often inappropriate to the context, and almost never answer any of the questions made to the patient. The patient could mouth words such as "pain" over and over again in a close-to catatonic state of mind.

A patient unable to pronounce words, but who still produces some sort of sounds with his mouth, is given a +2 value. The patient may be howling in pain, speaking in syllables, or just mouthing nonsense. If the patient seems able to understand he's being spoken to, but nothing coherent or intelligible comes out of his mouth when he tries to answer, this is indicative of an injury in the brain's cortex, specifically the parietal lobes. In any case, this is a sign of a very serious condition.

If the patient doesn't produce any sounds at all, he receives a +1 in the scale. These patients don't answer when they're spoken to and don't speak on their own. This condition is similar to the last condition in the eyes factor.

Motor

This is the last step of the scale, and it evaluates the motor response of the patient. It's as easy to evaluate as the previous ones, sometimes even easier than the verbal aspect. However, the terminology may be confusing to beginners, so it's important to state clearly what these terms mean.

The best condition a patient can be in is when they're able to follow simple instructions. This means that they're in control of their motricity, as well as able to understand language and create an appropriate response. Following instructions means a +6 in the value of the scale.

The following condition is when the patients limit themselves to point at their injury or pain. This shouldn't be confused with a patient asked to point at where it hurts and able to follow that simple instruction. That would mean the patient is in the highest condition, with a +6 in the scale. The patients who localize their pain are those with their arms right over the place that hurts them. A patient suffering a heart attack will probably get his hands towards his chest, for example. If the patient doesn't follow simple instructions, and instead he remains with his hands over the place that hurts him, he gets a +5 in the scale. This also applies to patients who immediately get their hands over a place that hurts them.

A patient that flexes his body and limbs to get away from the pain receives a value of +4. This is called normal flexion. It's the movement you'd expect someone to make if they were to get away from the pain. You have to make sure that the movement is fast, and it makes sense so that you don't confuse it with the next category. There shall be no extra movements that seem out of place and with no clear purpose.

A patient that flexes his body and limbs erratically is exhibiting and abnormal flexion, and thus, receives +3. This movement tends to be slower, and not every part of the patient's body is flexing to get away from the pain. There will be extra movements, such as an abdominal crunch or a leg extension. Another way to differentiate an abnormal flexion from a normal flexion is that the patient usually keeps his arm away from his body during a normal flexion. Unlike this, a patient with an abnormal flexion will usually get his arm over his torso.

When we stimulate a patient with pain and his body doesn't react with flexion, but by extending the limbs, that's an extension to the pain. These patients get a value of +2 on the scale. This movement makes no sense as a reaction to pain because it gets the patient's arm closer to the source of harm.

A patient that doesn't make any movements will always get a value of +1 in the scale. Some traumatized patients may be lying still on the floor and still react in some way to a stimulus. This category is for patients that don't react even if they receive a painful stimulus.

Measuring the Scale

Once you understand what each of the categories means, you should know the basic steps to follow if you want to measure the Glasgow Coma Scale the right way. There's a basic order you should always follow, as well as some tips for the stimulus.

You should start by checking the patient's current situation. Make sure that the patient isn't suffering from any condition that renders him unable to show a response to the stimuli. An intubated patient can't give a verbal response, for example, and that doesn't mean he should have a value of +1 in the verbal aspect of the scale. That only means that the scale can't be applied faithfully at that particular moment. These situations will produce a low value on the scale, but it doesn't mean that the patient is actually in dire conditions. Other measurements should be applied to assess the condition of the patient.

The second step is applied through observation. By observing the patient, you should also be able to grade many of the characteristics in the scale. A patient who opens his eyes spontaneously, speaks coherently, and seems able to move without issues can be assessed without interacting with him. This patient already has +4 in the eyes value of the scale. The patient also has +5 in the verbal value and +6 in the motor value; you can get a general idea out of this, but you need to work further in order to confirm this.

The third step is getting in contact with the patient and evaluating his response to stimuli. For this, you need to give the patient verbal stimuli, as well as painful stimuli. The spoken stimuli should always be used to assess orientation, as well as obtain basic information from the patient. Paramedics always ask the name of the patient, whether or not he knows where he is, and what day is it. If he's able to answer all of this correctly, he gets a +5 on the verbal scale. If he makes a mistake while answering this, he gets +4 on the scale because he's confused, and so on. You can also measure the eye's value with the verbal stimuli. If the patient has his eyes closed and only opens them when he's spoken to, then he gets a +3 in the eyes scale. If he doesn't open his eyes even when he's spoken to, he'll probably get a +2 in the scale. The remaining possible conditions will be evaluated with the other stimuli.

A simple order will be the next stimuli needed to assess the patient. Asking the patient to show them where it hurts, or point at the place of the accident, or do any other simple motor action will evaluate the first condition of the motor scale. If the patient is able to do this, he gets a +6 on that scale. By this point, a patient in good condition has already been evaluated correctly. The clinician gauged a +4 in the eye scale through observation; also, a +5 and +6 in the remaining scales through simple verbal stimuli. This should take no longer than eight seconds if done correctly, and time is valuable when you're trying to help these patients.

The last kind of stimulus is painful stimuli. This is often done at the same time as verbal stimuli because it saves time. A patient in good condition shouldn't need this; painful stimuli will only be needed to create a response on those patients who're not at or near the top of the scale. However, since you can't always tell for sure at first glance whether a patient is in good condition or not, the best course of action is to apply the stimuli anyway. There are two main maneuvers you should learn to apply if you want to assess a patient in bad conditions. You should cause pain on the subject over the upper half of his torso. This could be either by placing your knuckles over the patient's sternum and pressing down while sliding the knuckles or by pinching the patient's trapezius (the muscle that runs between the patient's shoulder and his neck). The reaction you expect is for the patient to bring his hand towards the pain. This counts as localizing the pain, and if the patient's unable to follow simple instructions, localizing the pain will give him a +5 on the scale. The other maneuver is to apply pressure on one of the patient's fingertips by squeezing them between your fingers. This will cause the patient to either flex his arm at his elbow rapidly and normally, flex it abnormally, or extend his arm at his elbow. If the patient's unable to follow simple instructions and feel localized pain, then this will give you the rating of the patient's motor response, either +4, +3, or +2, respectively.

The fourth and last step in the measurement of the Glasgow Coma Scale is to give each of the scale's aspects a rating and add the points to get a total value. The scale's rating goes from 3 (if the patient is in the worst condition possible) to 15 (a patient in the best condition). By consensus, 13 to 15 may be considered a mild head injury, 9 to 12 a moderate head injury, and 3 to 8 is a severe head injury. However, this scale should be considered a continuum rather than individual categories. Patients with scores of 3 to 5 have extremely poor outcomes. These patients are very likely not to survive, and during an emergency, if the paramedics must choose between trying to save these patients or a patient in critical condition and a better possible outcome, they'll prioritize the other patients. Traumatized patients with a scale of 6 to 8 need aggressive treatment, but they still have a far better possible outcome than those lower than that value. In any case, all patients with a value lower than 14 will need transportation to a trauma center as soon as possible.

The Glasgow Coma Scale is universally recognized and used because of its value to predict the patient's outcomes. It's also extremely useful for emergencies because it takes less than ten seconds to apply for any trained clinician and paramedic. Study the different conditions, values, and learn how to evaluate them, and you'll get it in no time.

Pulse Rate

Pulse rate is a vital sign that measures heartbeats. It's not part of the ATLS algorithm of the patient's assessment and treatment, but it still provides valuable information for the paramedics, as well as the health professionals involved in the treatment and recovery of the patient. The pulse rate is the number of times the blood is pumped through the arteries per minute. Since the blood is pumped with every heartbeat, it's a reliable way to measure the patient's heart beats per minute, which is called a heart rate. The normal heart rate goes from sixty to ninety heartbeats per minute. Higher than that is called tachycardia, and lower is bradycardia. However, some sources only consider tachycardia when the heart rate reaches over 100 beats per second, and bradycardia when it reaches under 50 beats per second. A patient under physical or mental health will probably have an accelerated heart rate, even tachycardia. Unless it reaches extremely high values, you shouldn't worry about it too much. The really worrying condition is a traumatized patient with bradycardia. In a concept similar to hypotension, bradycardia happens when the heart is unable to work correctly.

Measuring the Pulse

Many gadgets will help you with this easy task. If you use an automatic blood pressure monitor, you'll likely get a reading of the pulse rate as an additional value. There's another device that'll give you an automatic reading of the pulse rate, and it's called the oximeter.

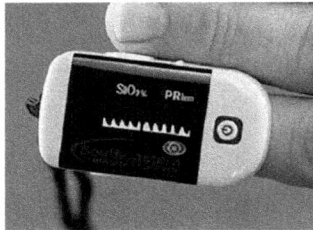

These devices are mainly used to measure oxygen saturation in the blood. This is particularly useful for patients with severe respiratory conditions such as pneumonia. However, oxygen saturation is not what we're looking for when we use an oximeter in a traumatized patient. We want to know the pulse rate, also indicated by the device. When you're building your first aid kit, you should always include one of these. It'll make the assessment of the patient much easier.

If you don't have an oximeter or an automatic blood pressure monitor that'll give you a reading of the patient's blood pulse, you must learn how to take the pulse rate yourself. It's simple enough once you understand the anatomy and the techniques behind it.

The right technique to measure pulse is by using your index, middle, and ring fingers. You can't use your thumb because it has a very noticeable pulse, so you could confuse your own pulse rate with the patient's pulse rate and gather a wrong reading. You should place these three fingers over the artery you're aiming for. The ring finger is used to press over the artery to suppress the pulse, and then release the pressure to allow the blood flow. This helps beginners feel the pulse, but it's not needed once you're proficient in this technique. You can stop using your ring finger once you're confident in your skills to localize and feel the patient's pulse. There are many places to feel the pulse, but the easiest ones to locate are the radial pulse and the carotid pulse.

The radial pulse is found at the end of the forearm, right below the hand, beside the thumb. It's between the radius, and the middle of the forearm, just like the picture. It's easy to feel a pulse there because the radial artery is right next to the skin (more details in chapter two). It may take some practice at first, but once you understand where it's located, it'll come easily.

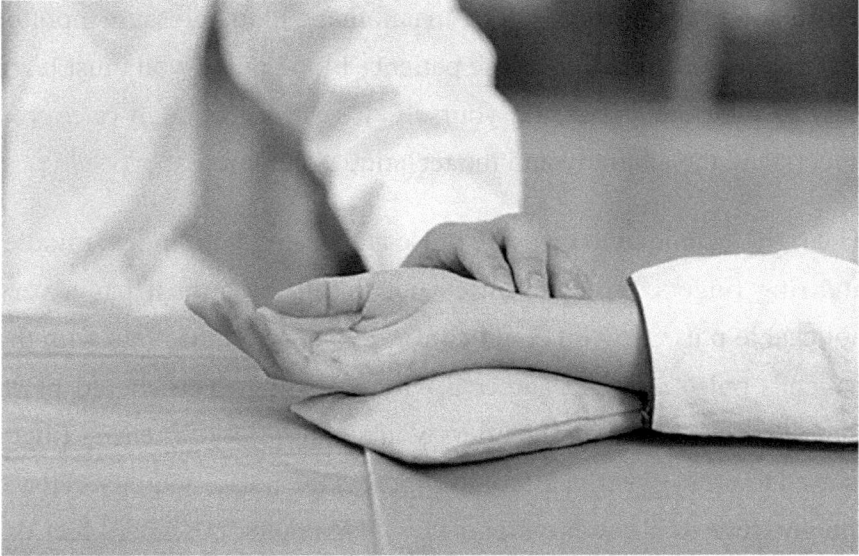

The second easiest pulse to measure is the carotid pulse. It's located in the frontal part of the neck, right below the chin, next to the Adam's apple, and slightly over it. This pulse is slightly harder to locate and feel than the radial pulse, so you may need to shift your fingers slowly until you feel it. Since it's less comfortable to the patient, and harder to find, people usually go for the radial pulse first. However, if there's an injury compromising the arm's blood flow, or if the patient's blood pressure is too low, it may be easier to assess the pulse rate in the carotid pulse because when the body's blood pressure is too low, the system prioritizes carrying blood to the brain, so the carotid pulse will be the last one to be affected when there's a hemorrhage.

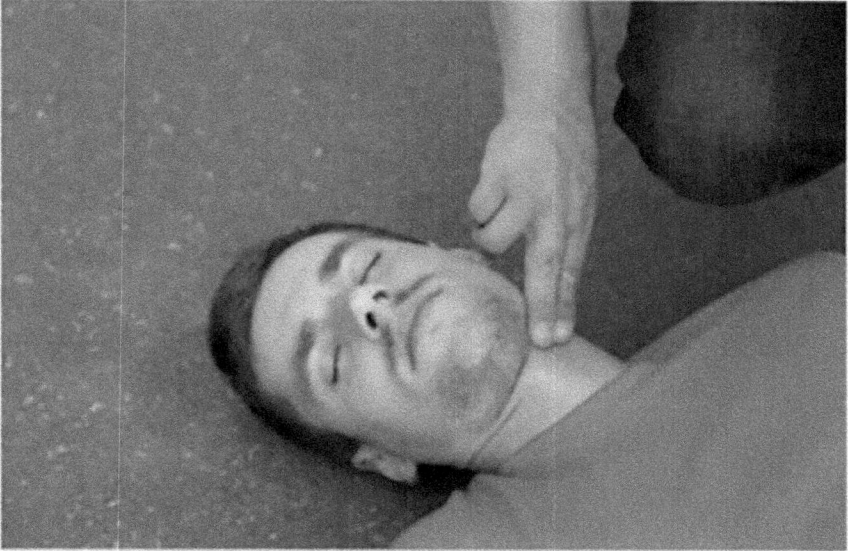

You can practice these techniques with yourself until you master them. We're all capable of taking our own pulse rates if we understand how to do it. Once you find your pulse, count the pulsations during a lapse of sixty seconds to get your pulse rate. Just like with the respiratory rate, this is the most reliable way to measure a pulse rate, but it's not fit for an emergency. Since one of your main concerns during an emergency should be to measure the pulse as quickly as possible, you could count the pulsations for fifteen seconds and multiply that number by four to get the patient's pulse rate. This is only possible if the pulse is regular.

If the pulse is irregular and you notice it's accelerating and decelerating constantly, you should count the pulsations for sixty seconds to get an accurate measure. Actually, if the pulse is irregular, this will also affect any electronic devices designed to measure the pulse rate. You'll see the numbers go up and down constantly as the pulse rate accelerates and decelerates, so in this case, you'll need to check the pulse manually. If the patient has a pulseless extremity, that is, a limb in which it's impossible to measure the pulse, this is a critical sign that tells us the patient needs to get treatment in a trauma center as soon as possible.

If everything's done correctly and there are no conditions that change the pulse rate of the patient, you should get a reading in about twenty seconds. Professionals used to this will take the pulse rate while they're taking the respiratory rate. This takes practice, but once you master it, it'll save you a lot of time, increasing the possibilities to save a life.

Note: If you're in a life-threatening or emergency medical situation, seek medical assistance immediately.

Chapter 8

Searching for Wounds and Triage

During the first approach to a patient, it's important to search for every possible wound. Considering the erratic nature of bullets, the injuries caused by them could leave an entrance and an exit wound that are completely apart from each other. Finding these wounds and treating them is a standard step in any first aid scheme. Also, if multiple patients need the clinician's help and it's impossible to treat them all, patients must be prioritized in order to treat and transport those who need it the most.

From Head to Toe

A head to toe assessment is a search and diagnosis scheme in which the clinician uncovers the whole body to search for any possible wounds. A pair of scissors or sharp blade must be used to get rid of the clothing and uncover the body. This is the only way to search efficiently for wounds and other injuries.

During the head to toe assessment of a gunshot wounded patient, some wounds require specialized attention. These wounds mean that the patient must be transported to a trauma center as soon as possible.

The wounds that should alarm the clinician and demand specialized trauma treatment are:

- Skull fractures

- Penetrating wounds to the torso, neck, or head. Penetrating wounds to the arms and legs also fall in this category as long as they're proximal to the elbows and knees.

- Instability and/or deformity of the chest wall

- Pelvic fracture

- Paralysis

Either of these means that the patient will need a team of health-care professionals specialized in trauma.

Triage

During the initial assessment, the clinician must identify those patients who need critical attention. This process is important because these patients can't be transported to any hospital but a certified trauma center. The sorting of patients between those who need immediate and critical attention and those in better conditions is called a Triage. The information collected during the initial assessment is of utmost importance for the patient, and it shall be gathered to aid the hospital staff in the treatment process.

Sometimes, a clinician or a paramedic must make the hard decision of letting go of a patient to give another patient a chance of survival.

Considering the ethical implications of these decisions, the process has been universally systematized to create an algorithm of choice-making.

The triage is based on assessing the patients and placing them in different categories. These categories have been illustrated by colors to be easily followed and understood universally. The idea behind the use of colors is to give the patients a mark according to their status. This tells the physician the condition of the patient even before he meets them. The colors used are the following:

Black

Patients considered in the black category are patients who are dead or almost dead. These patients can't be saved even if they receive treatment, or their chance to recover is so minimal that it isn't worth the effort if there's someone else who needs the treatment more. These patients are identified as unconscious patients that aren't breathing and/or their heart's not beating. They're clinically impossible to differentiate from a dead patient.

Red

Critical patients who could be saved if they receive medical treatment are placed in the red category. The patient's circulatory and respiratory systems are severely compromised. These patients are the top priority of the triage system.

Yellow

These are the patients that could wait at least 55-60 minutes to receive medical treatment. They've suffered injuries that may compromise the systems of the body, but their vital signs are normal.

Green

Green patients are those who can wait for several hours without receiving treatment. They've not received an injury to any of the systems of the body, and their vital signs are normal.

Chapter 9

Tactical Combat Casualty Care

The first approach of an injured patient has a predetermined structure in first aid. Paramedics follow the ABCD scheme of treatment as a general rule for traumatized patients. This work system starts with the Airways by making sure that there's nothing obstructing the airflow to the lungs. Then you have Breathing, where they check the breathing of the patient. Next, there's Circulation, vital sign assessment, and care for the heart. Then they finish their primary approach with Deficit, where they measure the neuronal deficit and condition of the patient. This primary approach is fit for patients under general circumstances, especially for patients who've suffered an accident. However, there's a better scheme to approach patients with a gunshot wound, the tactical combat casualty care system, or TCCC.

Also known as the "T Triple C," the Marines developed the tactical combat casualty care system as a system to treat soldiers who've received a gunshot wound. Instead of the ABCD, it follows a system called the MARCH(E) as a step-by-step walkthrough.

Massive Hemorrhage

The techniques used to stop a massive hemorrhage have already been described in this book (more details in chapter 6). As we've mentioned earlier, massive bleeding is the main cause of death in gunshot wounded patients. You should apply direct wound pressure, wound packing, and tourniquets if they're needed. If you don't have your equipment and bandages ready at the time you approach the wounded patient, you should start by stopping the bleeding by any means necessary. Use your fingers, palms, even your elbows if they stop the bleeding while you get your gauze bandages and get ready to perform any of the correct techniques. It's important to point out that you should never get your bare fingers in contact with a wound, to avoid contamination of the wound and protect yourself from any possible infections. A patient can die within minutes of massive hemorrhage is not addressed and treated, so the first step when you approach a gunshot wounded patients, is to stop the bleeding. There are five general steps used in the TCCC to treat massive hemorrhages.

Body Positioning

Placing the bleeding segment of the body above the level of the heart will reduce the amount of blood flowing towards it, therefore reducing the bleeding. This can only be done when the gunshot wound is in one of the extremities. Gunshots to the torso or the neck can't be elevated. Also, it's important to point out that elevating healthy limbs won't help improve the patient's situation; on the contrary; it'll make the bleeding worse. This is a technique used for patients with hypotension, and it would be helpful as long as there's no bleeding. However, if you elevate the legs of a gunshot wounded patient, you'll increase the blood returning to the heart and towards the place of the injury, increasing the bleeding.

Apply Pressure

The next step in the TCCC framework is to apply pressure over the wound. This is done as described in chapter six of this book. All wounds, no matter where they're placed, will go through this step. Gunshot wounds to the neck will only go this far in the framework, and the pressure can't be released until the patient is received by the specialized trauma personal in the health center.

Wound Packing

The next step is to apply wound packing. This will be done to almost every gunshot wounds, especially those large enough to fit many gauzes. The exception to this rule is when there's a gunshot wound to the neck; this is because wound packing could close the airways by putting pressure over the larynx or trachea. This is the step where you use a hemostatic agent, such as a combat gauze. It should be the first bandage you use in the process of wound packing. If the wound is located in the neck, then you must use the hemostatic agent during the previous step.

Pressure Bandage

Once wound packing has been applied, the next step is to seal the wound by applying a compression bandage. This is necessary for the patient's transportation since it allows him to be moved and manipulated without needing to hold the packing in place. For patients with gunshot wounds to the neck, this isn't needed either.

Application of Tourniquets

If there's a massive gunshot wound in one of the limbs and there is too much bleeding, the next step is to apply a tourniquet. Most people who die from a bleeding limb do so because the tourniquet hasn't been applied adequately, so it's important to make sure that the tourniquet is working and the bleeding stops.

Airway

The next step in the TCCC system is to secure the airflow to the body. Patients able to scream or communicate verbally are breathing correctly, and their airways are open. It's harder to assess this on unconscious patients, so the clinician must get close to the nose and assess whether they're breathing or not. If there's no risk of spinal injury, or a proper spinal immobilization has been placed, the patient could be rolled to a side to prevent him from choking with his own tongue. In the TCCC, the standard procedure to make sure the airway is clear is to insert a nasopharyngeal tube. **This can ONLY be done by trained medical professionals with proper equipment! This has been added for general information purposes only.**

Nasopharyngeal tubes are flexible rubber tubes used to create an artificial airway when the natural airway is at risk of being obstructed. The clinician must push the tube into one of the nostrils. Once the tube reaches the nasopharynx (the connection between the nasal cavity and the pharynx), it'll start going down the pharynx until it reaches the larynx. According to the TCCC, the only function of the tube is to keep the airway from getting obstructed; nonetheless, it doesn't hurt to get the tube into the trachea to secure an alternative airway.

There are a couple of situations in which a nasopharyngeal tube shouldn't be used. If there's severe trauma to the nose or nasal cavity, a nasopharyngeal tube can't be placed. Also, if the clinician suspects a fracture of the skull, central facial fractures, traumatic brain injury, or if the patient has any coagulation disorders, the nasopharyngeal tube can't be placed.

Respiration

Once the airway is secured, the following step in the TCCC system is breathing or respiration. This is the step where the respiratory rate is measured (more details in chapter seven). In the case of a gunshot wounded patient, this means evaluating the thorax and abdomen to see if there are any penetrating wounds and if the thorax is expanding symmetrically during respiration. If there's a penetrating wound to the thorax or even the abdomen above the belly button, then the clinician must consider the possibility of a pneumothorax. If one of the sides of the thorax is expanding more than the other one, then the clinician should also consider a pneumothorax, especially if the patient is having trouble breathing. These are all signs of either pneumothorax or tension pneumothorax.

If the patient has a penetrating wound to the thorax, air could be flowing into the pleural cavity every time the patient exhales while not being able to leave when the patient inhales. This causes a pneumothorax and, if left unattended, will collapse the patient's lungs. The way to avoid or treat a pneumothorax is by applying an occlusive bandage. Chest seals are the best fit for this, however, if there's no chest seal available, foil, credit cards, or anything strong enough may also be used. The way to apply an occlusive bandage is by placing it over the chest wound and using surgical tape to seal three out of the four borders of the bandage. This creates a "one-way valve" that won't allow the air to leak into the pleural cavity, only to leak out of it. If the patient's breathing is better after the application of the occlusive bandage, then the technique is working. However, if the breathing gets worse, that means that the air wasn't just leaking into the pleural cavity. It was also leaking out of a pierced lung and into the pleural cavity, once again, unable to leave the thorax fast enough. This is called a tension pneumothorax, and it must be treated by a surgeon. So, if the occlusive bandage deteriorates the patient's conditions after three or four minutes, it's imperative to remove chest seal off and get the patient to a health center as soon as possible.

Circulation

The fourth step of the TCCC system is the assessment of the condition of the circulatory system. This is the step where the clinician must measure the pulse rate and the systolic blood pressure (more details in chapter seven). If the patient's heart is growing weaker, that means that he'd lost an important amount of blood. This requires a transfusion of either blood or blood components. A professional paramedic or physician must do either of these, so there's nothing else to be done in a first aid environment before professional help gets to the patient. The only thing that could be done is to prevent more blood from leaving the patient's body by stopping the bleeding. If the patient's vital signs are deteriorating rapidly, there's a massive hemorrhage still taking place. This hemorrhage could be internal, in which case there's nothing else to be done until the patient receives professional help. It could also be external, in which case it's important to search for other wounds, or check if the wound packing and tourniquets are being effective and reinforce them if not. Remember to search for exit wounds as these may be hidden and could because of the hemorrhage that's deteriorating the patient's condition. The final consequence of massive hemorrhage is the cardiopulmonary arrest, in which case the patient's heart will stop beating, and the patient will need CPR (more details in chapter five).

Head Injury & Hypothermia

In the TCCC system, the H stands for both hypothermia and head injury. In the case of head injury, there's little to be done before the professional help arrives. It's important to remember to keep the cervical spine immobilized. Also, cerebrospinal fluid may leak out of the patient's nose and ears. This happens because of the swelling of the brain, and it can't be stopped. This kind of bleeding must be left alone to allow the brain to relieve its pressure. This is also the step to assess the Glasgow Coma Scale (or reassess if it has been evaluated earlier).

Hypothermia is also avoided during this step. It's a common consequence of a meaningful loss of blood since there's less blood to warm the body. If the clinician allows the patient's temperature to drop down, the body will waste energy trying to keep the temperature up. This is the reason why hypothermia is dealt with in the TCCC system. Covering the patient with a space blanket, a wool blanket, or any other clothing will help the body stay warm.

Everything Else & Evacuation

Once the previous steps have been taken care of, all immediate threats to the patient's life have been dealt with. Now the clinician deals with the minor wounds and prepares the patient for being transported to a health center. Minor bleeding wounds are treated with bandages, either by applying pressure and wound packing or just applying pressure. Then, any necessary immobilizations that haven't been done up to this point should be applied to prepare the patient for transportation more details in chapter six). If the patient is already properly immobilized when the professional paramedics reach him, then they won't have to waste so much time before transporting him to a health center. If there are no professional paramedics available, and the clinician is the one in charge of getting the patient to a health center, this is done after all immobilizations are in place unless there's a major threat to the patient's life that can't be addressed at the site (such as tension pneumothorax or a rapidly deteriorating neurological condition).

Note: If you're in a life-threatening or emergency medical situation, seek medical assistance immediately.

Chapter 10

The Mindset of a Rescuer

By this point, you have most of the required knowledge to treat a gunshot wound if the opportunity presents. However, knowledge isn't everything. It's imperative to have the right mindset in these critical situations. If you can't stay in control, there's the chance that you'll be overwhelmed by everything going on around you. This is absolutely normal, and it happens to everyone. Most paramedics and physicians suffer from a lack of confidence and are unable to perform correctly the first times they're in an emergency. Their amateur mindsets usually render them unreliable. The health system deals with this by not leaving them alone at all. None of them ever have to face these circumstances alone during training. Even when they join the workforce, they always have help during their first steps. Sadly, this is not a luxury you'll have. If you ever see yourself in a situation where you must treat a gunshot wound, it'll be because there's no one else around to help you. You'll have to take the reins of the emergency, so you must be mentally prepared for it.

Breathe

Facing an emergency can be mentally stressful and excruciating. Many things are happening at the same time that demand your immediate attention, which can be overwhelming. You have someone in front of you who demands your immediate help to survive. As if this wasn't enough to occupy your mind completely, you may also have to deal with other people, as well as a generally dire and dangerous situation. These factors can be overwhelming, and if you're not prepared, you're likely going to freeze over the action and waste valuable seconds trying to collect yourself. The best advice you can get in these situations is to breathe. If you ever feel overwhelmed in the face of this stressful situation, take a moment to breathe and count to three. By doing this, you'll give yourself the chance to adapt to what's to come. You get your mind in perspective, ready to rush over to the aid of those injured patients. It's better to spend six to eight seconds, collecting yourself than to spend the whole time stuttering and making mistakes. The best professionals use this advice, so don't feel ashamed if you need to stop and breathe in order to become useful; this is just part of the process of saving a life.

Take Charge

As the only person around with knowledge of how to treat a patient's injury, you should always be in charge of the whole situation. It's no good to treat a patient with care and haste if the situation around you is still a disaster, and people are crowding over you. It doesn't matter who you are or how you look like, everyone understands a good voice of command; it's in our nature. Also, you'll often need the collaboration of those around you, and you won't get any valuable help if the people aren't in the right mindset to help you. By taking charge of the situation, you'll be able to clear the way from those who're hindering your work, get the information you need regarding the situation, and even make them help you by bringing valuable tools. Some people are natural leaders; for them, taking charge of a situation is just a daily task. Some others have more trouble with this because they may be shy, or just not used to being on command. However, there are two tips regarding this advice that you can take if you haven't developed leadership skills in your life.

Fake it Until You Make It

This may sound cliché, but it's true, and it's backed with science. The mind is a very powerful tool, and we can trick it to get the results we want. If you've taught yourself during your whole life that you aren't usually the center of attention, likely, you won't feel comfortable in these situations. However, this perception of yourself can be changed, starting with your actions and growing from there. It doesn't matter if you think that you're not fit for leadership; fake it as if you were playing a part in a play. Behave like you'd expect a leader in charge to behave; this will allow you to act up to the situation, even if you're not used or comfortable with it.

After a while behaving this way, you'll be used to this. Your mind will learn that, contrary to your former beliefs, you're the type of person who takes charge of situations easily. It'll become natural for you, even if you don't consciously believe it yourself. If you want to be ready for the circumstances, if they ever come, of treating someone injured, all you need to do is give yourself the time to get used to this idea. Practice taking charge in your daily life to trick your mind into believing that this is the kind of person you are. You may practice this at work, at home, or even playing sports and games. You're building yourself to be the kind of person that's really useful under these circumstances. This is what those with gunshot wounds really need, so it's worth it to make an effort.

Learn from Others

You can see examples of leadership in your lives and all around the media. When you think about a leader who takes charge, you probably have a clear picture in your mind of someone who embodies this. See the way they act whenever they're the center of attention and use it as an example. It's not wrong to learn leadership from your own role models. It's a very primal skill, so it's universal, and it applies to everyone the same way. Pay attention to their attitudes and practice some of them to learn how to take charge of situations.

Believe in Yourself

It's easier to take charge of a situation if you're confident about your own skills and proficiency. If you feel like your knowledge is scarce, or your skills may not be good enough, it's hard to get people to follow you and take orders from you. There are a couple of things that you need to understand regarding this issue.

Your Mind is Not an Open Window

First of all, people are never aware of their actual level of skills and proficiency. They can't look straight into your mind and realize how much you actually know, or how well you're trained regarding anything. Of course, if you never take the time to practice, and don't take the part of studying these themes seriously, it'll show. Nevertheless, if you're proficient enough and you understand how to do what needs to be done, people won't realize this is only the first time you're treating a wounded person. This is especially the case if you do it with confidence, so don't worry about people doubting you in the midst of treating a patient.

The Value of Positivity

Secondly, you can tackle this issue with a good attitude and positive reinforcements. The same way that you can teach yourself you're the kind of person who takes charge of situations, you can also learn that you're good enough. The mind, as we've already stated, is a very powerful tool. By bombarding your mind with positive thoughts and messages, you can teach it to think and feel the way you need it to. Start each day, repeating positive sentences about yourself. Cover your room with post-it notes filled with encouraging messages. Don't underestimate the power of positivity to change your mind and your life.

The Imposter Syndrome

Thirdly, understand that not believing in yourself happens to everyone. This sort of thinking happens to every step of the professional ladder. People with titles, PHDs, and years of experience can also feel like they're not good enough, and this is clearly in their heads. This mindset is called the "imposter syndrome," and it's not limited to beginners. It's as if these people think that they're not worth their titles, as if they're an imposter around the rest of their peers. So keep in mind that, just as you're dealing with these doubts about yourself, so those everyone else. It has nothing to do with your actual level of skill and proficiency, so don't use it as a true way to assess your skills and build your self-trust.

Making a Real Effort

And last, you should still hone your skills and study until you're confident. This tip is down here because it seems to be obvious, not because it's less important. It's actually the cornerstone of self-confidence, as well as many other vital aspects of treating an injured patient. Your self-confidence and trust will feed and grow over your efforts. By studying and practicing, you'll teach your mind to expect great results from you. You'll start feeling like the kind of person who's able and proficient in what you do. Of course, studying and practicing is also vital if you ever want to be able to save a life, so there's no reason not to make a real effort about this. Study hard enough that you don't have trouble remembering anything, and feel confident every time you practice your skills, and your self-confidence and trust will be right there with you.

There's also another great aspect of our mind, and it's the power behind our reward system. Whenever we reach a goal we set for ourselves, no matter how small, it's still a reason for your mind to celebrate. It produces a rush of happiness and creates confidence in ourselves. So, as you advance in your studies, building trust in yourself will be almost automatic. All you'll need to do is work hard, pay attention to your results, and your mind will build your self-trust.

Don't Think Too Far Ahead

It's almost impossible to save a life if you spend most of the time worrying about it. When you face an injured patient, there's no real way to know whether they'll make it or not. The consequences are uncertain because there are too many factors in play, and most of them aren't evident without the help of proper tests. What this means to say is that there's no real way to make sure someone's life will be saved or not. Physicians and paramedics, especially experienced ones, already understand and embrace this concept. They focus on the job they have to do during an emergency, without thinking about whether they'll save a life or not. The job itself becomes almost mechanic. They follow the simple steps they know that they must take in order to save a life. This is the mindset you have to embrace during the treatment of an injured patient. There'll be time to worry later, but your mind has to be completely engaged during the process. Practice this concept and understand it if you want to be of any value to those who may need you.

Critical Thinking

It never hurts to be prepared, but sometimes life doesn't match our expectations, and we end up facing circumstances we're not prepared for. If you don't have the means necessary to do a correct immobilization, not enough gauze bandages to pack a wound the right way, or you lack any of the other required supplements of a good first aid kit, then you have to think fast and make the best of your current situations. You have to make difficult decisions if you don't have other alternatives. This mindset is called critical thinking, and it's about acting in spite of dire circumstances in an emergency.

It's ideal to be prepared to keep a patient alive while also giving him a better chance of recovery, but if you have to choose, the first one is always better than the last one. Some consequences, such as cervical spine injury because of a bad transportation technique, are way too dangerous to be treated lightly. These consequences can't be overlooked as long as you know, there's the possibility of professional help on the way. Nonetheless, you may have to make the decision of risking these consequences to save a life.

Conclusion

Our main goal as a species is survival and life preservation. Learning how to save lives isn't just a noble pursuit; it's wired into our genetic code as deeply as our need to eat, rest, and procreate. The human body is extremely complex, and the number of things that could go wrong because of a gunshot wound is too large to search for simple and generalized solutions. Therefore, if we wish to be able to preserve the life of someone who has been shot, we must be ready for it.

This book holds the basic knowledge to improve the survival chance of a gunshot injured patient. You, as a reader, need to prepare mentally to apply this knowledge. Study the material of the book, search for other means such as videos and other media to help clarify anything you have trouble with, and get it into practice. We can't know for sure whether we'll have to save someone who's been shot, neither can we control the exact circumstances in which this could happen; all that we can do is prepare ourselves for the possibility.

Preparing for disaster isn't limited to studying the human body and honing your skills; you also have to prepare a first aid kit to help you in this endeavor. You already must have a list of all the things you'll need. The combat gauze and the CPR drugs are probably going to raise the cost of your kit, especially because they have to be renewed constantly; however, they'll greatly increase the chance of survival of your patient.

The first chapter of this book may be designed as a walkthrough for someone who needs to prepare quickly, or worse, explains the steps out loud so someone else can use the knowledge to save someone without ever reading this book; however, that's not the best use of it. That chapter works best as a step-by-step reminder if you've already read it, the same way that this book works best if you take the time to study it and use it to prepare yourself. Make your life easier by preparing the best first aid kit you can have and memorizing the steps. When you consider the expected reward of saving a life, perhaps even someone you care about, no expense is too high, and no effort is too much.

www.ingramcontent.com/pod-product-compliance
Lightning Source LLC
Chambersburg PA
CBHW062111020426
42335CB00013B/921